Multiple Sclerosis
A Guide for the Newly Diagnosed

Multiple Sclerosis

A Guide for the Newly Diagnosed

Nancy J. Holland, RN, Ed.D.
Vice President, Client & Community Services
National Multiple Sclerosis Society
New York, New York

T. Jock Murray, M.D.
Director, Dalhousie Multiple Sclerosis Research Unit
Halifax, Nova Scotia

Stephen C. Reingold, Ph.D.
Vice President, Research and Medical Programs
National Multiple Sclerosis Society
New York, New York

demos vermande

Demos Vermande, 386 Park Avenue South, New York, New York 10016

Library of Congress Cataloging-in-Publication Data
Holland, Nancy J.
    Multiple sclerosis : a guide for the newly diagnosed / Nancy J.
Holland, T. Jock Murray, Stephen C. Reingold.
        p.   cm.
    Includes bibliographical references and index.
    ISBN 1-888799-06-4
    1. Multiple sclerosis—Popular works.   I. Murray, T. Jock
II. Reingold, Stephen Charles, 1948–   . III. Title.
RC377.H65   1996
616.8'34—dc20   96-35928
                                   CIP

Made in the United States of America

Dedication

Those diagnosed with multiple sclerosis today owe a great debt of gratitude to Labe C. Scheinberg, M.D. He opposed the voices who proclaimed defeat when faced with a diagnosis of multiple sclerosis, and insisted that much could be done to promote a productive and satisfying life, while limiting the negative impact of the disease.

Dr. Scheinberg is the champion of those with MS, from diagnosis throughout the disease course. He is the inspirational leader whose vision shaped this book.

Acknowledgments

Special thanks to Pamela Cavallo, MSW, Rosalind Kalb, Ph.D., and Cathy Carlson for their review and helpful critique of several chapters, and to our publisher, Dr. Diana M. Schneider, and editor, Joan Wolk, for their invaluable input and steady support throughout the project.

Contents

Foreword

The diagnosis of multiple sclerosis poses potential concerns related to all aspects of life and plans for the future. Family members and other loved ones are similarly concerned, and everyone involved struggles to make sense of life with this permanent intruder. One of the first responses is usually an active search for information about the disease itself and its potential long-term effects.

Most people diagnosed with MS have a good prognosis and will never have serious disability, yet there has never been a basic comprehensive discussion of the disease designed specifically for the needs of people who face the prospect of dealing with this chronic disorder. I have encouraged the authors of *Multiple Sclerosis: A Guide for the Newly Diagnosed* to write this excellent volume, which so successfully fills the need for information that addresses the specific issues of those newly diagnosed in an insightful and sensitive way.

This book appears at a particularly exciting time in the history of the management of multiple sclerosis. Never before has there been so positive an outlook for the future, as the result of research that has led to the development of new treatments designed to prevent progression of the disease and that hold out the hope of that most elusive target, a cure for what was previously regarded as incurable. At the same time, there have been major advances in managing the symptoms of the disease in a way that minimizes their impact on daily life and on the development of disability.

The authors discuss the nature of multiple sclerosis and what treatments are available, and provide practical guidelines for living, working, and coping with the disorder. This is followed by discussions of ongoing research and clinical trials that provide information needed to make decisions relating to new treatments. The need for information about the disease is addressed by a review of services provided by the National Multiple Sclerosis Society, a basic glossary of terms widely used in the MS literature, and suggested additional readings.

I am pleased to recommend this excellent volume to everyone who has recently received a diagnosis of multiple sclerosis.

Labe C. Scheinberg, M.D.
Professor Emeritus of Neurology
Albert Einstein College of Medicine
New York, New York

1

What Is Multiple Sclerosis and How Is It Diagnosed?

ALMOST ONE HUNDRED AND SEVENTY-FIVE YEARS AGO, physicians and pathologists described a chronic neurologic disorder associated with scattered patches of scarring in the central nervous system (CNS)—the brain and spinal cord. The name *multiple sclerosis* comes from the "sclerosed" or hardened plaques of scar tissue located at "multiple" sites throughout the central nervous system. Nerve fibers in the CNS are covered with a myelin sheath (white matter), which provides an insulating function similar to that of the rubber coating around electrical wires. Plaques damage the myelin around the nerve, and disrupt transmission of messages that communicate the desired action from the brain (message center) through the spinal cord, to various parts of the body. An example is a signal from the brain to the legs to walk. Patients with changes indicating impaired function of the CNS often have a clinical story of episodes of neurologic symptoms related to involvement of multiple areas of the spinal cord and brain.

In the mid-1860s, Professor Jean Martin Charcot at the Hôpital Salpétrière in Paris first described MS and its damage (lesions or plaques) in the brain and spinal cord in relation to the symptoms that separate MS from other diseases. He clearly defined the problems of MS and named the disease "sclérose en plaques," the name still used for MS in French-speaking countries.

Under the microscope the patches or plaques are seen as areas where the insulation (myelin) that normally surrounds nerve fibers (axons) is disrupted. There is an inflammatory reaction in these plaques, with some repair of fibers in older plaques, and some scarring in very old plaques. More episodes and more plaques may appear as years pass. Although repair can still occur and may often be almost complete, the repeated myelin breakdown, incomplete repair, and accumulation of scarring lead to the clinical appearance of progression in most of the people with MS.

Once the disease was described and had a name, it was possible for physicians everywhere to recognize it. It became clear that multiple sclerosis was not uncommon, but was in fact the most common serious neurologic disease in young adults. It followed a number of different patterns and courses, sometimes appeared more than once in the same family, and was more common in certain parts of the world and in Caucasian people.

As the physicians and researchers of today seek answers and learn more about multiple sclerosis, they uncover more questions and more things to learn. But we *are* learning more, there are more researchers working on the problem, and more research dollars are directed to solving it than ever before.

What Happens in Attacks of MS?

We have defined multiple sclerosis as a neurologic disorder characterized by scattered plaques of demyelination throughout the white matter of the central nervous system. Let's look in more detail at what those terms mean.

The multiple scars that give the disease its name are the end result of the patchy breakdown of the myelin cover, or "insulation," that surrounds nerves. Although the symptoms (numbness in a limb, blurred vision in one eye, or weakness in a leg) may suggest that one plaque has developed, there is probably more than one, possibly many. More surprisingly, some plaques may develop and heal without causing any symptoms.

At first there is an inflammatory response in the plaque, with cells present that are often seen in immunologic reactions. This has led to the belief that the episode of demyelination, or attack, may be an immunologic reaction of the body to some material, such as a protein, in the myelin sheath (see Chapter 2). Why this happens is uncertain. We know of other conditions in which the body's normal defense mechanism that reacts to "foreign" material seems to regard the normal proteins of the body as foreign and reacts against them.

When the episode of demyelination is settling down, other cells clean away the debris and remyelination, or repair of myelin, begins.

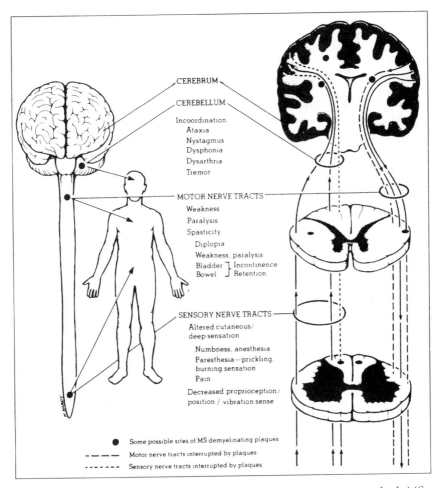

Figure 1-1. Diagram of the CNS, including all the principal regions in which MS lesions appear.

As a result, the symptoms that occurred during the episode of demyelination may improve or completely disappear, although some lingering damage may have resulted. However, the new myelin conducts nerve impulses somewhat more slowly than normal unaffected myelin. If a physician tests the speed of conduction in these nerves, they may be slower than normal nerves. This change has been used as the basis for developing tests to identify the disease, including visual evoked potentials, brainstem auditory evoked potentials, and sensory evoked potentials. These are electrodiagnostic tests that measure the time for a message such as a light seen by the eye to pass from the eye to the brain area for vision.

Episodes of demyelination accompanied by symptoms of MS may occur over many years. This is another hallmark of the disease—plaques that occur not only in multiple areas of the central nervous system, but also in multiple events over time.

The Course of Multiple Sclerosis

The course of MS varies from person to person. We do not know why one person has a progressive course of symptoms and problems, while another has mild disease that produces little disability throughout the life span. It can have different patterns in people in the same family, and what pattern a person has seems to have nothing to do with anything we can measure in their bodies, their life activities, or whatever steps they take to change things.

Despite this unpredictability, the course of MS can be classified into four common types recently defined by an international survey of MS experts:

- *Relapsing-Remitting*—This form of MS is characterized by clearly defined acute attacks with full recovery or with some remaining neurologic signs/symptoms and residual deficit upon recovery. The periods between disease relapses are characterized by a lack of disease progression.
- *Primary Progressive*—The disease shows progression of disability from its onset, without plateaus or remissions or with occasional plateaus and temporary minor improvements.
- *Secondary Progressive*—The disease begins with an initial relapsing-remitting course, followed by progression at a variable rate that may also include occasional relapses and minor remissions.

- *Progressive-Relapsing*—This pattern of MS shows progression from onset, but without clear acute relapses or remissions. It is more commonly seen in people who develop the disease after the age of 40.

In addition to these four major categories, some special patterns may occur:

- *Benign*—This term refers to a mild form of the disease in which the person remains fully functional in all neurologic systems 15 years after disease onset. This is the most difficult form of MS to "label" because it may require many years to see what pattern is developing. Many people with this form of the disease have mostly sensory symptoms or brain stem symptoms (vertigo, double vision, facial numbness).

- *Special Types*—Some disorders that initially involve demyelination limited to a specific area of the nervous system are considered to fall under the umbrella of MS since they may later involve the scattered demyelination characteristic of MS. Because not all of these people do have MS, their disorders are considered as separate disorders until more information is available, which may take many years. The two most common separate patterns are optic neuritis and transverse myelitis.

Remissions can occur at any time in the course of MS and can last for months or many years. Why they occur is unknown, and we are unable to tell in whom they will occur or when. They are more common in the early stages of the disease and in the relapsing-remitting type.

The Diagnosis of Multiple Sclerosis

It is often said that MS is a difficult diagnosis to make, but that is true only in some instances. Many patients who consult a neurologist can be diagnosed clinically without any doubt on the first visit. Other situations are more difficult, especially when a patient has minor complaints, shows no "findings" or abnormalities on examination, or has a symptom, such as numbness, that is also common in many other conditions, many of which are benign and transient.

The diagnosis of MS is made by a physician, often a neurologist, who takes a detailed history of the patient's symptoms and complaints, followed by a thorough physical and neurologic examination. Although the disease is suspected and ultimately diagnosed by the clinician's diagnostic skills, two things can assist in the diagnostic process.

The first is a set of criteria for establishing the diagnosis. Although the terms may sound very general, the patient suspected of having MS is classified by the physician as having "possible MS," "probable MS," or "definite MS." When a neurologist says that a person has definite MS, it means that he or she is in the usual age group for MS and has had more than one episode or attack of symptoms occurring in multiple areas of the white matter of the central nervous system (CNS); in some instances, instead of attacks, there will have been progression over a long time, again characterized by changes typical of involvement of many areas of the white matter in the CNS.

When a person does not demonstrate all the criteria for definite MS, he or she may be classified as having probable MS, on the basis that other conditions have been determined as unlikely, and additional features of the disease will become evident in time. Common examples of patients who are initially classified as having probable MS are those who present with their first symptom (thus it is not yet *multiple* in the number of episodes and not progressive over a long time) or those who have had repeated episodes but always in one site (thus not *multiple* in the areas involved).

The second helpful aid to the neurologist is a group of tests that may confirm the suspicion of MS. Remember, though, that the diagnosis is still a clinical decision, and there is no test that says definitively that MS is present. The test can only suggest changes that are compatible with the diagnosis, and the neurologist uses this to aid her or his clinical judgment. None are 100 percent accurate, but they are helpful in most cases.

Clinical Examination

The clinical examination has three major parts:

(1) *History.* The history includes not only the story of your symptoms and complaints, but also your general health during your lifetime, your operations and accidents, illnesses in your family, occupational information, and other details. This is often the most important part of the examination. The neurologist often makes the diagnosis during this part of the assessment, even before the neurologic examination or diagnostic tests, which are most often used to confirm the neurologist's suspicions from the history.

(2) *Examination.* To get a complete picture of your health and to better understand your symptoms, the neurologist carries out a *general physical examination* that includes listening to your chest and heart, taking your blood pressure, and examining your muscles and skin, as well as a *neurologic examination* that includes examining your eyes, the cranial nerves to your head and face, your strength, sensation and vibration over various parts of the body, your reflexes, and your balance and walking. Sometimes a patient is surprised to have his feet and abdomen examined when the complaint is of numbness in a hand. However, this overall exam provides a picture of the person's nervous system and is able to identify other conditions that might explain the symptoms he or she is experiencing.

(3) *Tests.* A number of tests can help to confirm that MS may be present and can also identify other problems that mimic the symptoms of MS. Some patients so clearly have MS when they are assessed that no tests are necessary, or only one may be used to confirm the disease and rule out other problems that might be under suspicion. Following are only the most commonly used and valuable tests.

Tests

MAGNETIC RESONANCE IMAGING (MRI)

A few decades ago the MRI would have seemed like science fiction—a test that produces a picture of your brain just by your lying inside a huge electromagnet that momentarily spins the molecules in your body. Minutes later the computer produces a remarkable picture of your nervous system that looks like a black and white photograph from an anatomy textbook. More remarkable for those who care for people with MS, the MRI is particularly good at detecting the patchy areas of change in the nervous system that occur with MS. It has become the most accurate and helpful test for MS, positive for changes consistent with MS in nine out of ten patients with proven MS.

MRI examinations are done while the patient lies on a table that moves inside a tube-like space in a large machine that holds a magnet. The person lies very still and the magnet sends information to a computer that receives thousands of tiny bits of information and uses them to generate pictures. These images are like slices or views at many levels throughout the brain or the spinal cord, or wherever the scanner is set. No discomfort is associated with the procedure, and the scanners are becoming faster, so that the length of time for a scan decreases each year. A few people have some feeling of claustrophobia and dislike the closed-in feeling of the narrow space. Most people can tolerate it, especially when they know how important it is and when they have a clear explanation of the procedure and receive support and encouragement from the staff. However, the acute discomfort experienced by many people can be easily reduced by mild sedation, such as Valium® 10 mg.

The MRI is an amazing technological advance that can help in the diagnosis of many diseases and is also helpful in research. However, there are some drawbacks to its completeness as a test for MS. Because it is so complex, the machinery, support systems, and personnel needed to operate them are very expensive. The cost of the test is often in the range of $500 to over $1,000, more if more complex procedures are necessary.

Another drawback is that it is not always positive in patients with MS, especially if they are at an early stage in their disease and have had only a few or very mild symptoms. Furthermore, the test does not "show MS"; it shows changes that could be *due* to MS. We must remember that occasionally other conditions cause similar changes. That is why the clinical picture is most helpful and can indicate whether other problems should be considered, or whether this is a typical story of MS symptoms, with typical findings of MS on examination, and with typical changes in keeping with MS on the MRI.

Finally, although the MRI can confirm the diagnosis, it does not tell us all the things you and we want to know, such as whether the disease is mild or advanced, or getting worse (those are clinical features). Further developments in MRI techniques will undoubtedly allow us to answer many more of these questions.

CEREBROSPINAL FLUID (CSF)

The cerebrospinal fluid (CSF) surrounds the brain and spinal cord and fills some cavities within the nervous system. A fine needle can be inserted into the low back (below the end of the spinal cord) to remove a sample of this clear fluid for examination of cells, protein, and electrolytes. If the radiologist wants to see the outline of the space in which the CSF flows, a *myelogram* is performed, in which a dye is injected into the spinal canal and an X-ray is taken. This procedure is done if compression of the cord by a disc or tumor is suspected.

A number of tests can be done on the CSF fluid, but the most useful in MS is to examine the proteins for the presence of *oligoclonal bands;* the protein is put on a gel and a current is passed through it in the laboratory to separate these bands. About nine out of ten patients with a well-established pattern of MS have bands in the CSF, but unfortunately this pattern is less common in early and very mild cases. The CSF is usually examined if the MRI is not helpful but the clinical picture is still suggestive of MS.

Many people have heard that having a lumbar puncture (also called an LP or spinal tap) is uncomfortable, but it usually does not cause much discomfort and can often be done on an outpatient basis. Unfortunately, about one third of people get a headache when they sit up after the test, a problem that may last for days. Lying flat on the abdomen to facilitate closure of the puncture site and abundant oral fluids to replace cerebrospinal fluid lost through testing should minimize this side effect.

EVOKED POTENTIAL STUDIES

The principle of evoked potential (EP) studies is simple. Nerves that have experienced demyelination conduct impulses more slowly than normal, even if they have healed and remyelinated. Evoked potential studies measure the rate and form of the impulse as it passes through specific nerves.

Visual evoked potential studies assess conduction of messages through the optic nerves behind the eye. To stimulate the visual system, the person may be asked to watch a TV screen that shows a checkerboard or some other pattern that rapidly changes, producing a stimulus that passes through the visual system to the occipital cortex of the brain (located at the back of the skull) where vision is organized. Electrodes over the scalp measure the wave form and the speed of the impulse to determine whether one differs from the other or if characteristic changes consistent with a diagnosis of MS are present.

The same idea can be adapted to the auditory or hearing nerve, in tests called *auditory evoked potentials* or *brainstem auditory evoked responses.* These tests involve listening to clicks in earphones while the wave form and speed of the nerve impulse is measured as it passes though the auditory nerve to the the brain area involved with hearing.

A third but less helpful variation is the *sensory evoked potential,* which measures the same conduction features when the skin is stimulated.

Watchful Waiting

Uncertainty is difficult to cope with, and many people would like answers to their problems, even if they are unpleasant. Definitive answers are not always possible.

In perhaps 10–15 percent of cases, the answer to the question, "Is MS the cause of these symptoms?" remains uncertain even after all available examinations and tests have been done. By this time the neurologist will have eliminated the possibility that other serious problems such as a tumor or a disc pressing on the nervous system are present. He or she often will know that MS *could be* causing the symptoms, but that other conditions might also be responsible. This uncertainty can be upsetting, but the approach at this point must be one of "wait and see," with periodic examinations and visits to the physician if new problems appear or changes occur. In most instances the diagnosis becomes clear over time. This requires patience by both the person with symptoms and the physician, but if they agree that they will wait *together* the patient usually accepts the situation, having being reassured about tumors and other worries. In some instances the problem later turns out to be something other than MS, often a mild, benign, or treatable condition. It is better to wait than to be prematurely labeled as having MS on the basis of unclear evidence.

The Outcome

When a person develops MS, he or she naturally wants to know what this will mean in the long term, relative to life, health, and family. Unfortunately, uncertainty and unpredictability are characteristics of the disease, as well as of its pattern of symptoms and course. What we can say in general terms is that the outlook is improving year by year and will continue to improve. Even before there was therapy to change the underlying disease, the life expectancy of people with MS had been extended to within the normal range as a result of the development of treatments such as antibiotics for bladder and kidney infections and better therapy for many of the complications of the disease. Newly available treatments for the underlying cause of the disease will undoubtedly change the long-term tendency for repeated attacks, progression, and disability, but we still have a long way to go. Research is proceeding rapidly, and although it will never be fast enough or great enough for those suffering daily with multiple sclerosis, we are heading in the right direction.

2

What Is the Cause of Multiple Sclerosis?

Introduction

MULTIPLE SCLEROSIS HAS BEEN KNOWN AND STUDIED AS A separate disease since the mid-1800s, but the cause of the disease (what scientists call the "etiology") remains a mystery. While many theories abound as to what the root cause of MS is, none has been proved. Because understanding what causes a disease can lead directly to a better sense of how to prevent and treat it, research into the etiology of MS is one of the most active areas of exploration. Recent findings have brought us closer to a complete understanding of MS and have led to new therapies and new approaches for future treatments.

Recent Theories About the Cause of MS

Multiple sclerosis appears as a neurologic disease (in other words, signs and symptoms of the disease can be attributed to problems in nervous system activity). Consequently, scientific work has focused on how nervous system problems in MS develop.

Autopsy studies of the bodies of individuals who had MS prior to death reveal the hallmarks of the disease in the central nervous system (CNS)—the brain and spinal cord. These include evidence of attack by the body's immune system, including inflammation or swelling of tissue, breakdown and loss of white matter or myelin surrounding nerve fibers, and appearance of hardened scars where myelin has been lost. Such immune system events cause a disruption of the proper flow of nerve signals from the brain and spinal cord to muscles and from sensory organs back to the brain and spinal cord, bringing about the typical neurologic problems in balance, gait, bladder and bowel control, numbness, pain, and others.

Many theories have been explored as to why the myelin of the CNS is attacked by a person's own immune system in MS. Some of these theories have been considered because they may explain a number of other nervous system diseases with some similarities to MS. For instance, congenital defects in nervous system structure or function have been considered, but there does not appear to be any direct link between abnormalities in MS and increased susceptibility to immune system attack. A direct effect of a virus or bacterial infection on nervous system myelin has been considered, since such infections can cause damage to the nervous system and do cause other nervous system diseases, but such direct effects do not seem to be involved in MS. Scientists have also considered the possibility that some environmental toxin or even a dietary imbalance may be the cause of MS. While toxic substances and diet can cause other nervous system problems, no research has supported such a cause for MS.

Although not currently popular as theories for the cause of MS, such ideas are still being explored by some scientists, and one often hears of "findings" suggesting that one or the other virus or chemical contaminant or heavy metal in the environment causes MS. In spite of the attention and excitement drawn to such "findings," further exploration has usually found the claims to have little if any scientific merit or relevance to MS.

A More Likely Possibility: Immune System Problems in MS

Research on the cause of MS since the mid-1950s has focused more closely on the possibility that MS may be a disease of immune system function that becomes clinically apparent in symptoms of the nervous system. Many scientists have focused their research efforts on the hypothesis that MS is an "autoimmune" disease, in which elements of immune function are misdirected and, instead of doing the normal job of defending our bodies against viral, bacterial, and parasitic infections, mistakenly turn against some part of the body—in this case against parts of the brain and spinal cord.

The concept of autoimmunity—a misdirected immune system attack—is by no means unique to MS. Diseases like rheumatoid arthritis, systemic lupus, juvenile onset diabetes, and others are also believed to be autoimmune in nature. Many of these share some important characteristics: cells or antibodies of the immune system attacking and destroying apparently normal parts of a person's body; a tendency to be more prevalent in women than men; possible treatment through routes that control immune function; and other similarities.

The evidence that the immune system is involved in MS is fairly clear, while the evidence that MS is an autoimmune disease is more indirect. First, people with MS seem to have clear-cut abnormalities in immune function compared to healthy individuals. These include, among other factors, evidence that specific white blood cells are primed to "recognize" and launch attacks against apparently normal components of the nervous system. In individuals with MS, there is clear reaction of white blood cells, called T cells, against proteins that compose CNS myelin. Interestingly, it has become clear since the mid-1990s that individuals without MS also have such T cells that react against myelin. A key difference may be that in those without MS, such damaging immune cells remain in the blood stream, separated from the CNS by a protective "blood-brain barrier" that prevents them from entering the nervous system and "seeing" central nervous system myelin. In MS, that blood-brain barrier is broken or breached, allowing the cells to flow into the CNS tissue and initiate their damaging effects.

Additionally, in individuals with MS there appears to be an over-representation of cells and other immune system components that enhance immune responses and a relative underrepresentation of cells and immune mediators that suppress immune responses. Most notably, in tissue from individuals with MS immune system cells are clearly found in active lesions of the brain and spinal cord. These immune characteristics are not seen in individuals who do not have MS.

While immune system involvement in MS seems clear, evidence that the immune problem is "autoimmune" is difficult to obtain in humans.

Actual proof of autoimmunity requires that immune system cells that react against normal body tissue and cause damage in one subject be injected into a healthy subject and cause damage and disease there as well. While this kind of experiment can be done in laboratory animals to prove autoimmunity, it is not possible to undertake such studies using humans with autoimmune disease and causing disease in otherwise healthy people.

For many years, one of the most important avenues of immunology research related to MS has come from study of a laboratory disease of rats, mice, guinea pigs, and primates, called experimental allergic encephalomyelitis (EAE), a disease that has been proven to be autoimmune. There are many similarities in clinical symptoms and CNS lesion patterns between EAE in these laboratory animals and MS in humans, and this has led most scientists to conclude that EAE and MS have similar involvement of the immune system. Thus, EAE serves in many regards as a "model" for the study of MS, lending credence to the belief that MS is likely autoimmune as well.

The Role of Genetics in MS

The possibility that MS may have a genetic component has been known for decades, based primarily on the fact that the disease sometimes "runs in families." We know that MS is not directly inherited, but it is increasingly clear that a complex set of genetic factors may help to determine who may be susceptible to MS and who may not.

Observations that suggest a genetic factor in MS come from studies of many populations around the world. It has long been known that there are ethnic or religious populations in the world that are genetically isolated (i.e., they rarely or never marry or bear children outside their own group, and thus have developed a relatively restricted and unique gene pool). Some of these groups rarely or never get MS. Examples include such religious sects as the Hutterites in Canada and such ethnic groups as Eastern European gypsies. While living in areas where there is a relatively high incidence of MS, these groups seem to be protected from MS.

Related to this is the fact that there are racial differences in MS. In North America, the disease occurs more commonly among Caucasians than among African-Americans, even in the same community. Multiple sclerosis is almost never is seen in Eskimos, even though the disease is quite common among Caucasian Canadians. In Africa, pure Bantus virtually never get MS, although Caucasians living in the same countries are susceptible. And MS is seen very rarely—and in a clinical type quite different from Caucasians—among Asians in the Far East and in immigrant populations in North America, Europe, and Australia.

Increasing evidence from families in which there are multiple cases of MS, either in a single generation or spread among several generations, has demonstrated an increased susceptibility or risk to developing MS in families where the disease already occurs. Perhaps as many as 20 percent of individuals with MS may have another family member—close or distant—with MS or with a disease that is likely MS but has not been correctly diagnosed. Results from a large-scale study in Canada indicate that the tendency for multiple cases of MS to occur in families is likely genetic and not due to any sort of shared environmental or dietary factor.

Even though there is clear increased family susceptibility, the risk of disease is still quite low. In the United States, about one in one thousand people have MS; when a family member (parent, sibling, aunt/uncle, etc.) has the disease already, the risk increases to 2–5/100, depending on the degree of relationship. This is an increased susceptibility, but still a relatively low risk. For twins, an important finding is that among nonidentical ("fraternal") twins, the risk resembles that for any other sibling; however, among identical twins (who are genetically identical) the risk of both having MS—being "concordant" for MS—if one twin has been diagnosed, rises dramatically to as high as 30 percent, a clear indication of the importance of genetic factors.

While such information might one day provide us with the ability to predict susceptibility, it cannot yet help us. The risk rates are low even within families where MS already exists. Inheritance patterns in MS are extremely complex and poorly understood. Large genetic studies have been initiated in several countries, most taking advantage of the existence of families with multiple individuals who have MS and many who do not. From these we have learned that there are many genetic factors that might contribute to MS susceptibility—it is surely not a case of a single gene defect, as has been shown for other diseases like Huntington's chorea and Duchenne muscular dystrophy.

The fact that identical twins are not always concordant for MS (i.e., the disease occurs in both twins) indicates clearly that, as important as genetic factors may be, there are other non-genetic factors that contribute to determining MS susceptibility.

What Sets Off the Disease? Possible Environmental Triggers

For decades studies of where MS exists in the world and where it is absent have suggested that there must be some triggering factor in the environment that starts the process. Data suggest that some factor—most likely infectious—must be encountered before the age of fifteen in order for the disease process to be triggered later in life. Although somewhat controversial, this finding stimulated the search, over the last forty-five years, for a virus that causes, or at least triggers, MS.

Many common and uncommon viruses have been proposed as causative agents for MS over the decades. Many of these proposals have been based on the presence of virus in tissues from individuals with MS or, more often, the presence of immune system antibodies against viruses in the blood. In each case further scientific work intended to confirm and expand upon data has failed to support the initial claim. In fact, it is generally believed now that individuals with MS have a heightened immune response against a host of common and uncommon viruses and that claims based on antibody responses against those viruses are likely very misleading. While this has not stopped the search for a specific MS virus, it has made such a search and any claims that have resulted subject to skepticism in recent years.

With a new understanding of the importance of immunology in the MS disease process, many scientists have shifted their view of the role of viruses and other infectious agents in MS away from the search for a direct cause of the disease toward finding out how an immune system response against an infectious agent may result in a later autoimmune disease. Increased attention has been paid to the possibility that many viruses (and perhaps bacteria and other pathogens as well) could serve as a trigger for the autoimmune process that becomes MS.

Demyelination: The Cause of Symptoms

The damage done by an immune reaction against myelin in brain and spinal cord might truly be considered the "cause" of MS, since it is this process that results in neurologic signs and symptoms observed in the clinic and experienced by the individual with MS. As noted previously, immune system T cells normally in the blood stream become activated against components of brain myelin. They cross the barrier between the blood stream and the CNS, causing local inflammation in the brain and spinal cord in scattered places—but most often around blood vessels and cavities in the brain called ventricles. This process eventually results in damage to the myelin insulation around nerve fibers. Lost myelin is extremely difficult for the nervous system to repair, and soon cells called astrocytes form scars where myelin previously existed.

Inflammation, loss of myelin, and scarring result in reduced conduction of nerve signals within the CNS, out to muscles, and back from sensory organs. These conduction problems produce the symptoms that characterize the disease.

So, What Is the Cause of MS?

Multiple sclerosis is, to be sure, a complex disease that is just beginning to be unraveled. There remains no known cause of MS, and it is likely that the disease is the result of a number of related factors. While symptoms come from problems in the nervous system, MS appears to be a disease of immune system function, most likely an autoimmune disease, that attacks the nervous system. Although not directly inherited, there is a clear genetic susceptibility. A triggering factor, or combination of factors, seems to be involved, but no definite virus or other infectious or environmental agent has been identified. The ultimate consequence of the immune system problems in MS is the entrance of immune cells into the CNS, attack of myelin around nerve fibers, and eventual myelin loss and scarring. The entire process results in the failure of nerve signals to operate properly.

3

What Treatment Is Available?

THE MEDICAL MANAGEMENT OF MULTIPLE SCLEROSIS IS
accomplished through a partnership of health professionals,
the person with MS, and his or her family. Aspects of both
symptomatic treatment and management of disease course
are addressed in this chapter.

People often say that there is no treatment for a disease
when there is no "magic bullet," a simple cure that makes
the disease go away, as penicillin may do for pneumonia.
There is yet no "cure" for MS, but there *are* many treatments
and approaches that help to manage the problems and
symptoms and to understand how to cope with the challenges, and there *are* many treatments and procedures that
reduce the symptoms of MS. Additionally, we are now
entering an era in which there will be agents that lessen the
number and severity of attacks, the progression of the disease, and the development of disability.

One of the most important first steps in dealing with
MS is to learn more about it. You need to know what you
can do to stay healthy and to reduce the problems that may
confront you and your family. *You* are in control of much

that is important in managing this disease. The fact that you are reading this book shows that you are already taking charge of one of the first things over which you have control—being informed and educated about MS.

Resources

Although your physician and other health care professionals will be able to offer many of the treatments and procedures discussed, you should begin by facilitating access to additional information through membership in the National (U.S.) or Canadian MS Society. Some people are reluctant to join at first because they are uncertain of the commitment that this implies. There is none. Being a member will provide access to the best up-to-date information as well as with issues and problems related to having MS. You can learn about ongoing research and important advances as they occur. Both MS Societies have many pamphlets on all important aspects of the disease (see Chapter 9).

There are many books about MS. Some are excellent, others are not. Some are by professionals who manage the disease, some are by individuals who have successfully adapted to limitations of the disease, and some are by enthusiasts for proposed new treatments. Consulting the MS Society will help to keep a balanced view since recommended publications are believed to be both accurate and helpful.

Since people with MS hear of many possible treatments from friends and the media, a useful resource is the book *Therapeutic Claims in Multiple Sclerosis: A Guide to Treatments*, prepared by the International Federation of Multiple Sclerosis Societies (Demos Vermande, 1996). This book lists over a hundred commonly used therapies for MS and indicates the rationale for their use, whether there is any evidence that they are helpful, and whether they are recommended. When someone tells you that vitamin B12, hyperbaric oxygen, or snake venom therapy is useful in MS, you can look up accurate information in this book (and you will find that none of these is helpful). You can also look up methylprednisolone, Betaseron®, Avonex®, and Copaxone® (and find that these are helpful).

Types of Treatment

Treatment in MS can be grouped under different categories of management:

- management of the acute attack;
- treatment of the underlying disease;
- management of symptoms.

Management of Acute Attacks

When there is a change in symptoms over a few days or weeks, with the development of new symptoms or the worsening of old ones, the event may be a new "attack" of the disease. It usually means that new patches of demyelination are occurring, in either new or old sites in the CNS. These are often mild and cease after a few days or weeks. Treatment may be indicated if the symptoms are severe or continue to worsen. The swelling and inflammation in the plaques of demyelination can be reduced by *high dose intravenous methylprednisolone.*

Some people may begin to recover soon after steroid therapy has started, but in others improvement may occur only slowly, even weeks after the treatment. As some spontaneous recovery is expected after most acute attacks, it is sometimes difficult to know how much was due to the treatment and how much would have occurred even without it.

Not all episodes of new symptoms need therapy with intravenous steroids, but a number of treatment schedules can be used if it is indicated. There are some differences in the total steroid dosage, the number of days of treatment, and the time between doses, but all are characterized by a high dose over a short period. This is usually given on an outpatient basis and is generally well-tolerated, although some people experience emotional changes during the therapy and may have trouble sleeping.

If there is numbness in a limb, dizziness, or some other symptom that is annoying but not limiting in any way, the neurologist may decide to *wait and see* if the problem clears spontaneously, as it often does. An attack that has stopped progressing and is improving may be allowed to clear on its own. High dose steroids help people to recover from an attack somewhat faster, but since they might recover just as well with time, decisions about treatment must be made on an individual basis.

Although it is reasonable to *rest* when you have MS, especially during attacks, it is generally overdone and overrecommended. There is good evidence that you will be tired if you do not get a reasonable amount of rest (although some tiredness in MS, referred to as "MS fatigue," does not respond well to rest), but there is little evidence that your MS will be worse with less rest. The fear that MS will become worse if you do not rest is without foundation and makes people fearful of doing normal things when they have symptoms. People may rest too much and thereby feel weary and weak, or stop work or neglect their responsibilities when they are capable of continuing these activities. This is based on the unfounded fear that MS will worsen without strict rest. A reasonable approach is to rest when tired and develop a schedule that allows a slower pace.

Advice to people with MS is *not* "rest, with reasonable activity," but it *is* "stay active, with reasonable rest." The difference is placement of the emphasis. Slow down and rest more when symptoms and fatigue are a problem or when an attack occurs, but stay as active as you can and increase your activity again when the symptoms settle down.

Treatment of the Underlying Disease

Only recently have there been therapies that hold promise of reducing the ultimate course of the disease. No therapies are yet available that stop the disease, but there are beginning steps toward more effective treatment, with medications that reduce the number and severity of attacks and result in less progression and disability over the years. The results are not dramatic, and most of these medications are very expensive, but they do represent an important step toward increasingly better therapy to halt disease progression.

BETA INTERFERON-1B (BETASERON®)

Beta interferon-1b was the first medication to be approved for treatment of the MS disease process. Interferons are naturally occurring proteins that are produced when the body reacts to a foreign substance such as a virus. Beta interferons seem to "calm" the immune system. The first studies of the drug were carried out on patients with relapsing-remitting MS and demonstrated a reduction in the number and severity of attacks, and a reduction of the number of lesions seen on the MRI brain scan. The drug is injected under the skin by the patient every second day, which is similar to the way a person with diabetes uses insulin. It does cause some side effects, which are usually tolerable. These include mild flu-like symptoms after the injections, which can be relieved by simple analgesics and lessen with time, and skin reactions at the injection sites, which may persist for days or weeks.

It is important to recognize that any of the new agents for MS help, but do not stop, problems or changes caused by MS. Some people who have taken them have greater expectations than the treatments can deliver, and become discouraged and stop the drugs when they continue to have further problems. The hope is that *over time* you will be better than if you did not have the treatment, not that you will suddenly notice yourself improving. It is too early to know how beneficial Betaseron® will be over the long term, but the first indications are that the benefits continue and may even increase over the years.

BETA INTERFERON 1-A (AVONEX®)

Beta interferon 1-a has also been shown to be safe and effective, and has the advantage that it can be injected weekly, although by a more difficult intramuscular injection. This medication has also been approved for the treatment of relapsing-remitting cases of MS. Completion of current trials will demonstrate whether the drug is helpful in other forms of the disease, and whether it is helpful in preventing the development of definite MS after an initial symptom that suggests risk for the disease.

GLATIRAMER ACETATE FOR INJECTION (COPAXONE®)

Glatiramer acetate is expected to be approved very soon for the treatment of MS, as it has also been shown to reduce the number of attacks and to reduce disability in the years it was studied in a clinical trial. It is taken by daily injection under the skin and is well-tolerated by most patients.

AZATHIOPRINE (IMURAN®)

Azathioprine has been available for many decades and has been widely used in Europe but less so in North America. There is some evidence that it reduces the number of attacks of MS and may reduce disability from the disease to some extent. It comes in pill form, is easy to use, and is inexpensive. However, there has been concern that this immunosuppressant might increase the incidence of certain malignancies (such as lymphomas) if it is taken on a long-term basis. Recent European studies have not shown such an increase, so its use is increasing. Regular blood tests are required when a patient is on this medication to detect early indications of liver dysfunction.

OTHER EXPERIMENTAL DRUGS

- There are promising early results with Cladribine (2-chlorodeoxyadenosine, 2-CdA), a drug that kills lymphocytes and has been used to treat lymphomas and certain types of leukemia. Several preliminary studies indicate that the drug reduces the progression of disability with less increase in lesion accumulation as indicated by MRI scans.
- Methotrexate prevents a model disease resembling MS (EAE) in laboratory animals and shows some ability to reduce the progression of disability in people with progressive MS.
- A classic method of inducing immunologic tolerance is through oral administration of the relevant antigens. Since MS involves an immunologic reaction against myelin, a logical approach is the oral administration of myelin. A multicenter trial of this is now under way, but no conclusive data are as yet available.
- Immunoglobulins are the antibody-containing fraction of human plasma. It has been suggested that artificially sustained high levels of circulating gamma globulin might block the harmful action of antibodies that are active in MS patients, such as those against myelin. The available data are conflicting as to whether intravenous immunoglobulin reduces the frequency of exacerbations in MS, and the results of properly controlled trials are awaited with interest.
- Roquinimex (Linomide®, quinoline-3-carboxamide) is an immunomodulatory drug that suppresses EAE. Preliminary trials showed a trend toward accumulation of less disability with linomide treatment, and a large multicenter trial in patients with relapsing-remitting and progressive disease is currently in progress; the results will be known in two to three years. The drug appears to be promising, especially because it has reduced the numbers of new lesions by MRI scan in controlled early pilot trials.
- Mitoxantrone (Novantron®)is an anticancer drug with immunosuppressive properties. It has proved highly effective in suppressing the animal model disease EAE, and encouraging results have been reported in several pilot trials, which showed a marked decrease in active MS lesions on MRI scanning. Controlled trials are under way in Europe, but their results have not yet been published.

Management of Symptoms

It is important to recognize that although a wide range of symptoms may occur with MS, a given individual may experience only some of them and never have others. Some symptoms may occur once, resolve, and never return. Because it is such an individual disease, it is not help-ful—and may be misleading and frightening—to compare yourself with someone else, who often will have different problems, a different pat-tern, and a different progression.

The most common symptoms of MS include numbness, fatigue, weakness, blurred vision, vertigo, poor balance, and difficulty walking. As mentioned previously, you may experience one or more of these and never have others.

MOBILITY

Weakness

It is common for a person with MS to have symptoms of weakness in one or both legs. Initially this may be transient, lasting days or weeks in an attack, but in some people weakness develops over many years as a major symptom. Because the nerves in the CNS have important func-tion in the motor control over muscles, patches of demyelination may affect these fibers and cause weakness in different muscle groups, most commonly in the legs. In some people, especially those who develop the disease after the age of 40, leg weakness and spasticity may be the only symptoms of MS, progressing slowly without any acute attacks.

It is common to develop weakness during an attack of MS, but some-times weakness may be present all the time. The pattern of weakness can be asymmetrical, involving one limb or one side more than the other, or it can seem to be only in the legs. If it comes on in an acute attack, it is treated with *intravenous steroids*. If it is a persistent feeling, it is impor-tant for the neurologist to decide how much is related to weakness in the muscles, how much is due to spasticity or increased tone in the mus-cles, and how much is contributed by a change in sensation that make the limbs seem more clumsy.

If weakness is present, you should be encouraged to increase your level of *exercise* to strengthen the muscles. A physical therapist can help if you experience a lot of weakness, but if the weakness is mild you can do an exercise program on your own. It is important to remember that any muscle can be strengthened. Just as "normal" muscles can be made stronger by exercise, weak ones can be trained and strengthened by exercise. The muscles may not return to normal but they will be stronger than they otherwise would have been, and that is always worthwhile.

If there is a lot of weakness in a limb, various aids may be necessary, such as an ankle brace for a drop foot or a cane to help with walking until improvement is seen. Foot drop is usually first noticed when "tripping" over your foot occurs, causing the tips of shoes on the affected side to become scraped or scuffed. If weakness persists after treatment with steroids, a referral for *physical therapy* may be arranged so that the problems can be assessed, an exercise program developed, and any immediate problems treated.

You should continue a regular exercise program even after weakness has improved (see "A Note About Exercise" later in this chapter).

SPASTICITY

A complex control of muscle movements normally allows some muscles to contract and some to relax when a movement is carried out. This control can inhibit certain muscles and contract others when there is disruption to nerves in the CNS, resulting in the simultaneous contraction of many muscles, both the ones that help (agonists) and those that oppose the movement (antagonists). This causes the "tone" to increase in all the muscles, the limb to feel tight, and the limb movements to be slower and less smooth. It is more work and more tiring to walk with legs that have spasticity.

Spasticity can be reduced by exercise and by normal use of the muscles. It is important to perform stretching exercises of the spastic, tight muscles to prevent contractures, a state in which the tight muscle shortens. Each muscle should be stretched fully and held for a minute. (See "A Note About Exercise.")

A number of medications that are considered muscle relaxants do not work well in MS and can have side effects. The most effective medication for spasticity and the symptoms that it produces (spasms, cramps, pain, aching), is baclofen (Lioresal®), which can be taken in different ways depending on the symptoms, their severity, and the person's tolerance to the medication. Because some people have painful spasms only at night and minor spasticity in the daytime, a nightly dose may be all that is needed. Others need relief from spasticity all the time, and a schedule of four doses a day is developed. Because all patients can reach a dosage level that seems too high, causing a general feeling of weakness and drowsiness, your doctor may start you with a very low dose, perhaps half a tablet (5 mg) twice a day, and slowly increase by adding a further half tablet every three days until symptoms are reasonably controlled. If symptoms are helped at a low dose, the dosage is held there. If a patient develops side effects when the dose is increased, these may be eliminated by skipping a dose and going back to the previous level. Baclofen is very helpful in reducing the spasms and pain sometimes associated with spasticity but is only somewhat helpful in improving function limited by spasticity.

Tizanidine (Zanaflex®) is an effective antispasticity agent that has effects similar to baclofen. It is especially effective for night spasms and is sometimes effective in reducing spasticity in patients who do not respond to other agents. Its use in combination with low doses of baclofen may produce an optimal antispasticity effect with fewer side effects. Tizanidine is less sedating than diazepam or baclofen.

Disturbances of Balance and Gait

Disturbances of gait and balance are common in MS because they can be affected by changes in different parts of the nervous system. A person may note that he or she does not walk or stand as steadily if experiencing incoordination, weakness in one or more limbs, numbness, dizziness, vertigo, or even visual problems. One of the most troublesome causes of gait disturbance is spasticity in the muscles of the legs. For some people, this is the most limiting problem of MS. Because so much of what we do involves being mobile, this problem causes the most disability and handicap in the disease over the lifetime of many (but not all) people with MS.

In many instances, difficulty in walking comes with the various symptoms of an attack of MS, improving or clearing as the attack settles down. In other instances, it is an ongoing problem. A person with MS may have few other problems except a gait difficulty that slowly increases over a period of years. This pattern is more common in those who develop the disease later in life.

Physical therapy can be helpful for gait difficulty, and a physical therapist can show you techniques of gait training, muscle strengthening, exercises, safety hints, and the use of aids.

A Note About Exercise

Exercise is important for everyone, especially a person with MS. One exercise program that you should do daily, or even more than once a day if your muscles are very stiff, is a program of range of motion exercises. Each joint is put through its full range of motion to keep it healthy and lubricated and to stretch and loosen the muscles that move the joints.

A simple exercise program that anyone can manage is the 10-10-20 exercise program, in which 10 general exercises are performed, each for 10 repetitions, for a duration of a 20-minute exercise period. The 10 exercises are general ones that improve overall fitness. They can be altered according to individual capacity and the need to overcome specific problems or weak areas. They can be individually designed by a physical therapist and modified as needs change.

Swimming has a number of advantages, although it is often more difficult to arrange on a regular basis. Swimming exercises most muscles, and some movements and exercises can be done better in water because the water supports the body during movement. The water should be cool since most people with MS are sensitive to heat and may be bothered by exercises that increase body heat or warm exercise rooms. Function may be improved just by the cooling in a swimming pool. Although swimming in the ocean can have the same effect, waves can easily put you off balance.

Relaxation techniques are useful and improve the enjoyment and rewards of a regular exercise program. They involve methods of learning positive relaxation of the mind and body, deep breathing, and mental imagery, combined with alternating contraction and relaxation of various muscles.

An exercise program should be *regular* and *enjoyable*. Anyone can carry out a boring exercise program for a few weeks, but not for a lifetime, which is what we all need. That is why many basements have a corner with almost new exercise equipment that has had little use. Some machines look terrific, but are not very enjoyable to use, and sometimes we think that it is the machines (or physiotherapists) that are going to make us strong. *YOU* do the exercises, not the machine.

Exercise programs that many people enjoy include swimming, mat exercises, walking, and Tai Chi, but you must think about the exercises that you would find most enjoyable and can imagine still doing regularly years from now.

SENSORY SYMPTOMS

Numbness

Numbness covers many alterations to the sensory system, affecting sensation, particularly in the skin. People may experience numbness, but more often they feel tingling, pins and needles, burning, coldness, or other sensations that are difficult to describe. The disruption to the sensory nerves can be in the spinal cord, the brain stem, or the brain itself.

Tingling and numbness are "normal" symptoms that virtually everyone has experienced (a leg falling "asleep," dental anesthesia, cold feet in the winter), but these common occurrences are due to pressure, anesthetics, or cold to a *peripheral nerve* in an arm or leg, whereas MS affects only the myelin of the nerves in the central nervous system. It may seem as if the nerve in the leg is affected in MS, but in fact the demyelination is in the *central nervous system*, not in the peripheral nervous system. Numbness is most often felt in the ends of the limbs, the feet and lower legs or the hands, but it can seem to rise from the legs up to the upper abdomen. Sometimes the numbness seems to have a level, as if a belt of numbness was wrapped around the abdomen; it also may be painful, with decreased sensation below the level.

Although numbness is often only a brief annoyance, it can cause other problems if it persists or if it only partially clears. You may drop things when your hands and fingertips are numb, even light objects such as paper, because you do not know how tightly you are gripping them. Because feeling in your fingers is decreased, you may need to use your vision to help you recognize things that you could identify previously with your fingertips. You may have trouble identifying objects in your purse or pocket because numbness can decrease your ability to recognize a comb or a coin by its characteristic feel. You may not realize that good balance involves sensing information about the muscles and tendons in the limbs, which is carried to the nervous system by sensory nerves. If numbness is present in the legs, people use their eyes to maintain good balance. They notice, however, that they look down a lot when they walk and have difficulty walking in the dark and over uneven ground.

Numbness is occasionally accompanied by disagreeable sensations (dysesthesias), such as burning, "creepy-crawly" feelings or sensitive skin (sensations similar to those felt when dental anesthesia is wearing off). These disagreeable feelings usually improve as sensation improves, but they sometimes require treatment. When numbness or dysesthesias occur as part of an acute attack, it usually improves with intravenous steroids. More persistent disagreeable sensations may be reduced by a tricyclic antidepressant such as amytriptyline (Elavil®). This medication is very effective in relieving sensory problems, even though depression is not related to these symptoms

Some sensation changes are described as pain, which is discussed later in this chapter.

Facial Numbness

A common and upsetting symptom in MS is numbness on one side of the face. This is a minor symptom, however, and usually clears without treatment. You might have a tingling feeling or a numbness, often described as similar to dental anesthesia, which can at times involve the gums and tongue. Symptoms around the face are perceived as more disturbing to people than the same degree of numbness elsewhere, such as the foot or hand, but in fact facial numbness often goes away in days or a few weeks. The neurologist may also find subtle differences to various sensations in the face, of which the person is unaware.

Vision Loss

Different types of vision problems may occur in MS. *Optic neuritis* (sometimes called retrobulbar neuritis) is an episode of demyelination in the optic nerve behind the eyeball. Because it occurs in the nerve, a physician looking in the eye during the first episode may not see anything wrong. Later some scarring may occur in the optic nerve and it will look pale in the back of the eye, seen by the doctor through a hand-held instrument called an ophthalmoscope. High dose intravenous steroids is the standard treatment when one eye or occasionally both eyes are affected. Symptoms include blurred vision, loss of peripheral or "side" vision, and one or more black or "blind" spots. Total loss of vision in one eye may occur in some instances. Optic neuritis sometimes also causes pain in the eye, which clears quickly when steroid treatment is begun. Vision returns more slowly. It is common for individuals with relapsing-remitting MS to have one or more episodes of optic neuritis, although many people never experience this problem.

Another visual complaint people with MS may experience is a vague feeling that their vision is not as clear as it should be, even if a recent eye examination indicates that vision is normal. The problem may be some trouble with certain contrasts in the visual fields, or with color, which causes a mild change that is not usually detected on standard eye tests. When this occurs, text with sharp contrast is easiest to read. An unusual symptom is a decrease in vision associated with exercise (Uthoff's phenomenon), probably due to an increase in body heat, which affects nerve conduction. Vision returns when the person stops exercising and cools down.

Some people with MS experience double vision and complain that they cannot see well. Actually, the vision in each eye separately may be normal, but the eyes do not focus together. Although it is annoying, double vision usually clears on its own or responds to intravenous steroids. It is rarely a persistent problem, and can be temporarily relieved by patching one eye.

Another problem in eye control that may be experienced as a visual problem is *nystagmus*. When a physician asks you to move your eyes in different directions, eye movements and control are being tested. Nystagmus is a regular fine jerkiness of the eyes that may occur when looking to the sides, which is usually not noticed by the patient. Sometimes the eyes operate differently in that situation, with one having more jerkiness than the other. This causes a sensation that the environment is moving (oscillopsia) or looks double when looking to the sides. In some people the pupillary response to light is slowed, experienced as difficulty with bright lights, especially while driving at night. Glasses with photosensitive lenses usually compensate for this problem.

All that affects vision is not MS, and the MS patient should have *regular eye examinations* to see if he or she needs glasses to correct the vision changes that occur in all of us.

Pain

In the past it was believed that pain was unusual in MS. We now know that pain in one form or another occurs in more than half of all people who have the disease. It may take the form of an aching in muscles, shooting pains, jabbing facial pain, or discomfort from burning, tingling, or other sensory changes. The first step is to determine the specific cause of the pain. Not all pain is the result of MS, so other problems must be considered. Since pain problems in MS have specific treatments, as does pain from other causes, it is important to identify the underlying cause.

The spasms and cramps in the large muscles of the legs that occur when tone is increased by spasticity can be reduced by physical therapy, exercise, relaxation techniques, passive stretching, massage, and local cold. The pain associated with spasticity can often be effectively reduced with baclofen (Lioresal®).

Remember that not all symptoms in people with MS are due to the disease and that any problems that cause pain in anyone else can also occur. Joint pain, back pain, abdominal pain, headaches, and other problems may be due to conditions that are not MS, and should be investigated and treated just as they would if MS were not present.

Facial Pain

A type of nerve pain that can occur in the face, called *trigeminal neuralgia*, is characterized by a sharp, jabbing, knife-like pain, usually over the cheek and sometimes over the eye on one side. Although it can occur as an isolated syndrome in the elderly, it often indicates the underlying demyelinating process of MS in a younger person. Several types of pain occur in the face, including temporomandibular joint (TMJ) pain, tension headache, and migraine. If trigeminal neuralgia is the cause, it is treated with a group of medications that decrease the nerve firing. The initial treatment is usually carbamazepine (Tegretol®), to which most people quickly respond well. In the few people who have unacceptable side effects, baclofen (Lioresal®) or diphenylhydantoin (Dilantin®) is substituted.

A small number of patients do not tolerate these medications, lose the beneficial drug effect, or do not respond to them. In such cases, a surgical procedure may be considered. It is usually done on an outpatient basis by a needle procedure through the face into the 5th nerve. This is usually successful. A more complicated neurosurgical procedure is directed at separating the nerve from a pulsating artery that irritates it, but this is more often seen in the elderly. The cause in the person with MS is the presence of a plaque in the connections of the 5th nerve in the brain stem. Although it can cause severe facial pain, trigeminal neuralgia is usually successfully managed. It is not uncommon for the problem to return months or years after it has been controlled, but treatment can be restarted if it does.

Hearing Changes

It is unusual for people with MS to notice any change in hearing, other than that seen in the normal population, but MS can on occasion cause a decrease in hearing. More commonly, a subtle change can be noted on specific testing of the hearing system, but without producing noticeable symptoms. Significant hearing change due to MS is rarely a problem, and when acute episodes of hearing loss occur, full recovery can be expected.

ELIMINATION

Bladder Control

The most common symptoms of bladder involvement in MS are the need to urinate *often* (frequency) and the need to urinate *now* (urgency). If these symptoms are particularly troublesome, involuntary wetting (incontinence) can occur because of difficulty getting to the bathroom in time. Many people manage this by being aware of their symptoms and taking opportunities to urinate regularly. Markedly restricting fluid intake, which seems to be a logical method of dealing with the problem, is actually a bad idea; your kidney and bladder systems need a continuous flow of fluids to excrete wastes and minimize the opportunity of infection.

If frequency and urgency are a more serious problem than you can manage by simple measures, medications such as oxybutynin chloride (Ditropan®), propantheline bromide (Probanthine®), or flavoxate hydrochloride (Urispas®) may control the problem, but it is important to determine that urinary retention is not present before these are initiated. A number of problems with the bladder can occur in MS, each of which needs a specific approach to management. If simple measures and these medications are not sufficient to control the problem, a urologic assessment is needed to see if other approaches are required.

It is important to know that bladder problems are common in MS, can be managed in most cases with simple measures, but can lead to serious complications if untreated. Urinary infection in men should always be explored further, and recurrent urinary infection in women also requires investigation. If burning or painful urination occur, especially when the urine has a foul odor and is cloudy, you probably have a bladder infection and need to be in touch with your physician right away.

Avoidance of bladder symptoms can be helped by drinking about eight glasses (eight ounce) of fluid daily, limiting citrus juices (orange, grapefruit, and tomato), and adding cranberry juice one or more times daily.

Bowel Control

Bowel control problems are less common than bladder problems, and in most cases they also can be managed by simple methods. The first step is to maintain a regular bowel schedule. Try to have a bowel movement each day after breakfast, as establishing a regular daily pattern avoids constipation and a tendency to irregular bowel movements as a result of inactivity. Your diet should be high in fiber, including a serving of bran each day. Drinking enough is also critical, as dry stool is the most common cause of constipation. Another factor in bowel health is exercise—this helps maintain good bowel function in everyone, but is especially important when you have MS.

OTHER SYMPTOMS

Fatigue

People with MS may notice two patterns of fatigue. One is a feeling of tiredness and weakness that occurs with increasing exercise or other physical activity. For instance, walking may be fine at the onset, but the legs may become increasingly heavy and tired after walking a long distance, with some dragging of the feet. Strength is recovered and the person can continue again after sitting down and resting for a brief time.

Another kind of fatigue is a general feeling of exhaustion, which can be more annoying and limiting. This can be mild or severe, intermittent or continuous. You may experience this type of fatigue quite suddenly during a normal day, with an abnormal fatigue coming over you like a wave, making it difficult to continue. More commonly, it is a general fatigue that is present no matter how much or how little you do. It may be aggravated by overdoing activity or getting less sleep, but may be present even if you do nothing and have had a good night's sleep. When we ask people with MS to list the symptoms that bother them the most, fatigue is usually at the top of the list. It is also the most common symptom experienced by people with MS.

Most people learn to modify their day in ways that allow them to manage fatigue, such as taking brief rests or even occasional naps. Others say that they cannot do this because of the nature of their work or responsibilities, and they push through the fatigue without its causing any problems. It simply makes you tired to overdo it when you have fatigue; it does not worsen your MS. The most common problem from overdoing things is to be more tired. It is common for people to say they can push through their work or task but that they pay for the next two days if they overdo it. Sometimes the fatigue will characteristically appear at about the same time of day, allowing for some restructuring of activities if your work or other schedules permit.

Most people with MS say that the fatigue they experience feels abnormal, unlike the normal tiredness that everyone experiences. Most neurologic diseases are not associated with this pattern of tiredness, although a number of other autoimmune diseases do exhibit this unusual fatigue. Because it is so "different" and so common in MS, it is surprising that it was not recognized as a characteristic symptom of MS until recently. By a serendipitous observation it was found that amantadine (Symmetrel®) taken twice a day is helpful in reducing fatigue in over half the people who experience it. Another medication that may be helpful is a mild stimulant, pemoline (Cylert®), which is taken once or twice a day.

Tremor

Everyone has some tremor (to see the normal physiologic tremor put a piece of paper on top of your outstretched hand). Multiple sclerosis may be accompanied by different types of tremor, which range from annoying to fairly disabling. There are a variety of approaches to controlling them, some of which people learn on their own. For instance, bracing the forearm against the side or on a hard surface reduces arm and hand tremor. Another variation is to have a method of immobilization that is used for some specific task such as writing, but is removed when the task is over. Physical and occupational therapists may use patterning, repeating movements to make them smoother and more automatic. Adding weights to the limb may reduce tremor. There is also adaptive equipment that can be useful.

Medication is only partially effective, and some of the drugs tried in the past seemed to give limited assistance and caused side effects. Perhaps the only drugs that may have a significant effect are beta blockers such as propranolol (Inderal®). Mild sedatives and tranquilizers may help, but they are probably only worthwhile when the person has some other need for a sedative, such as tension or anxiety, which aggravate tremor. Stereotactic surgery may be used in selected cases, but this is unusual and carries significant risk.

Vertigo

Vertigo is the sensation that many call "dizziness," but since that term can mean different things, it is necessary to explain exactly what you feel. Vertigo has the sensation of movement, whether it seems that the room is moving or turning or that you seem to be moving. If it is severe, the room seems to be spinning, or you may feel like you are tipping or falling or that the floor is coming up to meet you. This sensation usually is due to a disturbance in the vestibular system of the middle ear or its connections within the brainstem and brain. In MS the problem is most often in the nerve connections in the brainstem. It is usually transient, lasting hours or occasionally weeks; it is unusual for it to last much longer. If it persists, it can be treated by stimulating the vestibular system or suppressing the vestibular reflexes with medication.

If the onset of vertigo is acute and lasts for many days, it can be treated by intravenous steroids, but usually it settles by itself. When vertigo is worsened by movement, as it often is, paradoxically the problem can be reduced by purposely stimulating the vertigo. Thus *positional exercises* can be done using a simple method on a soft surface such as a bed. The vestibular system is stimulated by falling on the bed to one side three times (the vertigo lessens each time), then to the other side, then backwards. There is often a *position of comfort* when a person has vertigo, with fewer symptoms lying on one side and more on the other, and with the head supported at a certain angle. Sedatives are helpful, as is diazepam (Valium®), which suppresses the vestibular reflex.

Vertigo can be mild, experienced as a slight swimming feeling in the head. Mild nausea and poor concentration are often associated with this. Again, positional exercises and an exercise program are more helpful than sitting still, which is the natural tendency.

Seizures

Seizures are not common in MS but occur in approximately 5 percent of patients. They are usually effectively treated with common anticonvulsants such as phenytoin (Dilantin®) or carbamazepine (Tegretol®). An unusual type of "seizure" is a localized spasm that is more like a major muscle spasm than an epileptic seizure and often occurs on one side of the body. Such spasms also respond to medication such as carbamazepine.

Facial Weakness

Facial weakness can occur suddenly in MS, although it is uncommon. When it does happen, especially early in the course of the disease, it may resemble Bell's palsy, a benign form of acute facial palsy that often follows a viral infection. Both Bell's palsy and the facial weakness of MS respond to steroids. In MS no treatment may be needed if the weakness is mild or is already rapidly improving on its own.

Alternative and Complementary Therapies

For many centuries there has been an approach to curing and healing illness and symptoms that has been separate from the medical profession. At any time and in any century these have taken hundreds of forms. Some are common sense approaches that the "wisewomen" and elders in the community used to treat minor problems without the necessity of calling a doctor. Aside from these home remedies there are therapists who offer treatments that are outside the mainstream of medicine. These therapists include herbalists, psychic healers, reflexologists, homeopaths, naturopaths, and many other therapists who pursue an approach based on belief or ideology rather than a scientific approach based on questioning, testing, changing, and advancing.

Believers in alternative medicines usually do not want their beliefs tested. The treatment is not based on science or data, so they may argue that science is not an appropriate way to assess its value. This reaction against traditional ways of evaluating therapies complicates the ability of the medical community to sort out objective therapies from ineffective ones.

Some therapists offer methods that do make people *feel* better, including massage and other physical therapies, and that is good, but it should not be confused with a specific therapy that is claimed to cure MS or reduce MS disease activity. Therapies that impact general health fall within the "wellness" concept and are considered "complementary" rather than "alternative" measures.

Are alternative therapies safe? That depends. Many are safe and may even make people feel better. Other therapies, particularly remedies that are unapproved and unregulated and may contain mysterious and changing ingredients, can cause serious side effects and even death in some instances. Alternative therapies, home remedies, and herbal treatments are often thought to be safe because they are "natural," but that is not justified; many are not safe and many are not natural. There is often little information on their safety or benefit. People take such substances at their own risk. Some alternative medicines have made people very sick; they can also react with medications that are being taken for other reasons.

What are you to do when you hear from a friend, another person with MS, or the media that something may be a treatment for the disease? Talk to your physician. He or she will not mind discussing a newspaper clipping or other source of a "therapeutic claim." Your physician will be able to tell you the pros and cons of most therapies. Another helpful source is your local MS Society, which should have information on anything you have read or heard about. Finally, consult *Therapeutic Claims in Multiple Sclerosis: A Guide to Treatments* (see the resource list at the end of this book), which lists over one hundred of the most common therapies said to be useful in treating MS, explaining what each is about, what evidence there is for its use, and whether it is recommended.

In commenting on alternative therapies, we do not wish to be discouraging, but we *do* want people with MS to take only medications and therapies that have been demonstrated to be safe and effective. We recommend that you find evidence that this is the case before you try anything.

What Is Ahead in Research for New Treatments?

As described in Chapter 7, research is now progressing at a pace we have not seen before. It is natural to hope for a sudden "breakthrough" in MS, a discovery that will solve the problem, but this rarely occurs. More often research adds a new bit of knowledge that leads to the next questions, which, when answered, add still more knowledge and lead to more research and more answers. This eventually translates into better understanding, better treatment, and, hopefully, ways to prevent the disease. Hollywood may like stories about dramatic breakthroughs, but the world of research and medical advances is of one step leading to the next, eventually leading to the answers we are seeking. It is a long and painstaking process, but it is the way we advance.

People with MS and those who care for them are more hopeful than ever as we see improvements in care, new advances in neuroimaging and diagnosis, better control of symptoms, new medications that change the disease, and an increase in our understanding of the underlying genetic and environmental mechanisms in the disease. Just as people with MS have reason to hope, so do those of us who work to find the cause and cure of the disease, and to bring better care to those with MS and their families, and never before have we had such good reason to hope.

4

Practical Guidelines

THERE ARE MANY THINGS YOU CAN DO TO STAY AS HEALTHY
as possible, take control of your life, and cope with the challenges that multiple sclerosis may bring. The disease is not
in control of you—*you* are in control of your life, your attitudes, your relationships, your approach to problems, your
interests, and your activities. The best way to take control is
to obtain more information and learn more about MS.

This chapter discusses some things you should do and
some things you should not do. For example, you *should* get
more information about MS; you *should* make sure you have
an opportunity to ask questions about the disease; you
should exercise; you *should* try to live a normal, active life,
adapting to any limitations; you *should* work to improve
your relationships; you *should* express a positive attitude; and
you *should* have regular medical assessments.

The things you should *not* do are actually fewer. *Don't*
withdraw from life and friends; *don't* stop exercising; *don't*
expose yourself to hot environments; *don't* try every drug,
herb, therapy, and procedure that you hear about without
first getting reliable information about the scientific evidence, possible benefits, and side effects; and *don't* feel
ashamed or diminished because you have multiple sclerosis.

Should I Learn More About MS?

MULTIPLE SCLEROSIS IS A DISORDER OF THE CENTRAL NERVOUS SYSTEM. Many things are known about it, and many advances are being made. There are still many unanswered questions, but it is important to learn more about the questions that are being asked by researchers and the theories that are being tested.

The best initial source of information is the MS Society. In the United States, call 800-FIGHT-MS to reach the National MS Society, and in Canada 800-268-7582. See Chapter 9 for the number of the nearest office of the MS Society of Canada.

What Should Others Know About MS?

IT IS IMPORTANT FOR YOUR FAMILY, FRIENDS, AND COWORKERS TO UNDERSTAND MS. Initially you may feel that you do not want anyone to know that you have MS. That is understandable, but it is essential to tell the people you love, and others when necessary, so that they can understand and help you deal with the disease. Most people are pleased and surprised at how supportive and understanding others are when they are informed. Many people may have guessed that something was wrong, but did not know what to do or say. Until they know the truth (see Chapter 6), employers may not understand your need to take time off or to rest and may think you are not working well. Decisions to inform should be made on an individual basis, but in general disclosure is a good idea.

Once family and friends are aware of your diagnosis, they might benefit from literature that would allow them to better understand MS. In particular, your family should understand your symptoms and problems so they can be as helpful and supportive as possible. This is not possible if they are unaware of your MS and its specific impact on you.

Who Can Answer My Questions?

IT IS IMPORTANT TO HAVE YOUR CONCERNS ADDRESSED AND YOUR QUESTIONS answered. Sometimes people are afraid that they might ask too many questions or that their questions might not be clear. Make a list of the questions you want to ask. Call the MS Society, or bring the questions to your physician on your next visit. You will probably find that they are questions most people ask and that they are not new to the staff. If there is no clear answer to a question, it is important to find that out as well. Each new piece of information will add to your overall understanding of MS.

What Can I Learn from Other People Who Have MS?

PEOPLE WITH MS SOON LEARN THAT IT IS A COMMON NEUROLOGIC disorder and there are many others in their community who have the same disease. It often helps to talk to others who share the challenges and problems of coping with MS, but there are some cautions. You cannot compare yourself with others in terms of the type of disease, the course, or the symptoms. Multiple sclerosis is an individual disease, and you will probably find that the features of your MS are quite different from those of the next person. It may seem puzzling that there are so many individual patterns for the disease, but that is actually fairly common in other diseases as well. The variety of symptoms of MS is great, so the apparent variations in individuals seem great as well.

One way that people with MS can benefit from each other is in self-help or support groups. These take various forms, but they are usually small groups that meet in homes or in community facilities to talk about and better understand MS. The object is always to take a positive approach and to take control over everything that you can manage, so that you can help yourself and others. The MS Society has information on support groups, including how to join one or how to start one.

When Is Information Not Helpful?

MISINFORMATION IS NOT HELPFUL AND CAN CAUSE MUCH TROUBLE AND distress, not to mention wasted time and money. If someone says that mercury in dental fillings causes MS, check it out from those who know—staff at the MS Society, someone in the MS clinic in your area, or your physician—don't go to the dentist and have your fillings removed. If someone tells you that ginseng cures MS, check it out. If someone says there is a doctor in a clinic somewhere who has a cure for MS, call the MS Society, not your travel agent.

What About My Activities?

PEOPLE WITH MS SHOULD LEAD NORMAL AND ACTIVE LIVES WITHIN THE limitations of their symptoms. This means that we encourage activity more than rest, staying active and involved rather than withdrawing and dropping out. We want people to remain productive and working. It is understandable that symptoms and problems may make this harder for you, that doing things may take more time and energy, but it is still better to do it than not to do it.

ı   People with MS are happiest and at their best when they live normally and carry out the activities they enjoy. There are no absolute limitations—if you feel like climbing a mountain and do not have symptoms and problems that limit you, go for it! Unfortunately, MS does cause symptoms that may limit activities to some extent. It requires adjustment so that you can continue to do as much as you can, in the time you need, and in the way you can manage. If you work at managing your problems, coping with any limitations, and keeping a positive attitude, you can not only do many of the things in life you want to do, but you may also accomplish much more than others without MS, as they often do not use these positive skills to deal with life.

What About Exercise?

SIMPLY PUT, EXERCISE IS GOOD FOR EVERYONE. WHEN THE DIAGNOSIS of MS is made, you should set about getting yourself in the best shape that you can, both mentally and physically, in order to manage any challenges that come with the disease. We all benefit from regular exercise, and it is even more important for the person with MS. If fatigue is a problem, you should arrange your exercise for times when fatigue is less bothersome, schedule it in periods with breaks, or redesign the type and pattern of exercise so that you can still do it.

In general, the best exercise is one that you enjoy, so that you will still be doing it in six months. Exercise should be a lifetime habit for all of us, and this is true for people with MS, even if the exercise program needs to be modified at times. Decide what you like to do and would enjoy doing almost every day. Try to involve others in exercise as well. Exercise programs in the community have a tendency to motivate you to participate regularly; they also have an enjoyable social aspect.

Can I Overdo It?

IT WOULD SEEM LOGICAL TO BE CONCERNED THAT OVERDOING THINGS might cause attacks of MS and worsen the disease, and that we should rest and avoid strain and work. This is not good advice. There is no evidence that doing a lot, exercising, or even overdoing activities or physical exercise has any deleterious effect on MS. True, it may make you tired for the next day or so, but there is no evidence that it worsens your MS. Some patients "push through" their fatigue, which may make them tired the next day but does not harm them.

It might be tempting to blame overactivity for the development of a new attack of MS or a new symptom, especially if it happened a day or a few days later, but a careful accounting of strenuous events, stressful events, and the occurrence of attacks would show that this is probably coincidental. Don't worry about activity; be reasonable, keep active, and do what you can.

How Much Should I Rest?

Because fatigue is a major problem for many people with MS, a reasonable balance between maintaining your normal activities and taking brief rests is appropriate. People usually find their own balance of activity and rest, and in this way keep up their activity, work, and other responsibilities.

It is important to recognize that the fatigue in MS is not "normal" tiredness that follows too little sleep or a long hard day. The fatigue in MS is often an abnormal sensation; it is unrelated to the amount of sleep and activity and feels different. It can occur in waves and seem overwhelming at times. Adapting the level of activities is often successful, and some medications may also be helpful (see Chapter 3).

Do not rest too much. *Activity* is a more important watchword than rest in MS.

What About Stress?

All people experience stress in their lives. Being given a diagnosis of MS is stressful. Having to see yourself and your life in a different light, with greater uncertainty, is stressful. But marriage, raising children, doing our jobs, and the "dailyness of life" also bring stress. The central point is not whether stress is present in your life (it almost always is), but your response to it. People can, and do, react differently. Some see stress as a problem to be solved. Some respond emotionally, collapsing in tears, becoming depressed, or lashing out angrily at others. Some are initially upset, but then set about overcoming or dealing with the stress. Others do not believe it is possible to deal with it and give up. It is not the stress; it is our reaction to it that makes the difference.

When people react to stress in a nonproductive way, they often state that anyone would react the same way. That is not actually true, but they are unable to see any other way of reacting. Fortunately, by analyzing such events, you can learn how to react more positively. It is not easy and sometimes requires counseling, but a person who reacts ineffectively to stress can learn how to respond better. It does mean that you must recognize that your responses could be more productive before you can work at it or seek help.

Can I Develop Better Coping Skills?

WE ALL HAVE CERTAIN PATTERNS OF COPING. SOME OF US REACT MORE intellectually to problems and stresses, while others react more emotionally. Most of us have a combination of the two; it is the *balance* of intellectual problem-solving responses and emotional responses that is important.

It is natural to feel upset when something stressful happens. It is not normal for that to be the only response, however, and there is a point at which we must think clearly and objectively about what the stress is all about, how we can analyze it, and how we can most effectively deal with it. *That* is combining the appropriate emotional and problem-solving aspect. You can improve these coping skills by improving their components. When a stressful event has passed, you can analyze how well you responded: whether your emotional response was appropriate and balanced, and whether the steps you took were the most effective and efficient ones for solving or dealing with the problem. Such analysis often gives you a different perspective, particularly if it is done in an honest fashion and enables you to see how you could respond more effectively the next time.

How Can I Maintain a Positive Attitude?

THE MOST IMPORTANT FACTOR IN DEALING WITH MS (OR ANY CHALLENGE in life) is a mature, positive, and good-humored attitude whenever possible.

Some people struggle harder than others. There is no question that a positive attitude is of great importance, as a negative person cannot tolerate very much adversity. Multiple sclerosis does not make you positive or negative; you already had an approach to life before you developed the disease. MS can challenge your approach, your positivity, and your good humor, however, so it is important to make an even greater effort to overcome difficulties in a way that makes you feel good and improves your relationships. People like to be around those who are positive and good-humored. We can understand those who are negative and turn their frustration on others, but they don't manage well, are unhappier, and don't learn to take control of the things they can manage.

What About My Relationships?

Good relationships are helpful to all of us, and they become even more important when we have difficult challenges to deal with and overcome. One important aspect of taking control of your health and your future is to strengthen your relationships. It has a positive effect on you when you do everything you can to improve your relationships with your spouse, your children, your family, your friends, and everyone with whom you come in contact. It may seem simplistic, but it is actually one of the most important things you can do. Our relationships with others are central to our happiness and state of well-being, and it is rewarding to begin to improve them.

Should I Tell People I Have MS?

It is natural that you may have felt uncertain about telling people— even your family or close friends—when you first were told that you have MS. It is hard to recognize that something about yourself has changed, and it is worrisome to think that it may change relationships and how people regard you. Eventually you will come to recognize that you are still the same person, that the people who love you will continue to love you and support you, and that others are generally understanding and helpful. Sometimes they may try to be too helpful, as most people do not want the relationship to be altered or to be treated differently. All of these feelings, plus some embarrassment about "having an illness," make many people want to hide the diagnosis. They think "maybe if I pretend the problem doesn't exist, it won't exist."

It is a good rule to be honest and open in our relationships and interactions. Of course, like all health matters, the fact that you have MS is a private and confidential matter, so who you confide in is a personal issue. It is common to keep the information within a small circle initially, especially as everything may be calm and stable for many years. A problem begins to develop when symptoms cause difficulties that are visible to others, but they have not been made aware that you have a health problem. At that point others may wonder, worry, and speculate about what is happening, and their speculation can be more harmful than the truth.

It is also worth considering that people feel excluded and not trusted when they are kept in the dark yet know that something is being kept secret.

There are some instances when keeping a medical problem a secret can be a serious offense or can cause serious problems. You cannot lie about having a medical problem when answering questions on insurance forms or other official documents. There are only a few instances when it is proper to ask such questions, but in such instances you must answer truthfully.

What Happens When It Is Hot?

MOST PEOPLE WITH MS FIND THAT THEY ARE MORE HEAT-SENSITIVE. IT does not occur with everyone, but most people notice that they become weaker or dizzy, or even feel sick, in a hot bath, on a hot humid day, or in a warm environment. They also notice the opposite—they feel better and function better when it is cooler, when they are swimming in cool water, or when they move from a warm room to a cool one.

Remyelinated and partially damaged nerve fibers may function less well when body temperature is elevated and, conversely, the nerves function better when temperature is lowered. This tends to be a transient phenomenon and does not produce a lasting effect. However, it can produce marked weakness, and patients often describe themselves as feeling like a "dish rag" or "wiped out" on a hot day. This symptom was once the basis of the hot bath test, which was utilized as a test for MS before modern diagnostic tests were available. Although it is suggestive of MS, it is not accurate enough to be an important test.

You may wonder whether becoming weak in a hot environment will make you worse, but the phenomenon is transient and disappears as soon as you cool off. We do recommend that you avoid such environments because you will feel less well, function less well, and have more symptoms when it is very warm. Air conditioning is often required in summer months to maintain reasonable temperature control and is considered medically necessary for tax purposes (a letter from your phsyician is needed). Avoidance of sunbathing, saunas, and hot tubs is strongly advised.

Should I Change My Diet?

THE DIETARY APPROACH TO THE MANAGEMENT OF MS HAS A LONG HISTORY. It is difficult to perform clinical trials on diets, but there was interest and some suggestion of a positive response from studies of diets that are low in animal fats (essentially a low cholesterol diet) and with a supplement of a vegetable oil such as sunflower seed oil or evening primrose oil. A few of these studies showed some positive benefit; one large study showed no benefit. There was also some suggestion that people with early and mild disease benefit the most. Many people use the simple approach to diet of lowering the amount of animal fat and supplementing it with a vegetable oil because it is a healthy diet and everyone in the family would potentially benefit from such a diet. Many more complex diets have been recommended in MS, which have little logic or justification, and are so complicated that people give them up after a short time.

The most important point is to stick to a balanced, healthy diet, maintain normal weight, and limit your intake of animal fat. This is a good dietary recommendation for everyone.

Should I Sleep More?

HOW MUCH YOU SHOULD SLEEP IS BASED ON YOUR NORMAL PATTERN. SOME people require eight or nine hours a night, whereas others require five or six hours. The average is seven hours of sleep, and the measure of effectiveness is how rested you feel in the morning. You should not change your sleep pattern because you have MS. Since fatigue is a major problem for many people, there is a tendency to think that they will be less fatigued if they sleep more; even with normal or greater sleep hours, the person will still tend to feel tired during the day. Surprisingly, oversleeping often makes people feel more tired. It is worth remembering that many factors can decrease the quality of sleep, including alcohol and many drugs.

What If I Need Surgery?

THE ANSWER TO THIS QUESTION IS SIMPLE. IF YOU NEED SURGERY AND THERE are good indications for surgery, you should have it. If you do not need surgery, you should not have it. This is a good rule whether you have MS or not. There does not appear to be any increased risk to people with MS who undergo surgery. In the past there was concern that the stress of surgery might precipitate MS attacks, but the number of attacks of MS that occur in those circumstances is probably the same as that which would be expected in an average population of people with the disease, and no more. This relates to the previous point that there is little evidence that stressful events precipitate attacks of MS, whether they involve surgery, anesthesia, trauma, or major life events. The most important rule is to be assured that surgery is truly indicated and necessary. This rule is not different because you have MS.

Is Pregnancy a Risk?

THE OBSERVATIONS ABOUT MS AND PREGNANCY ARE NOW FAIRLY CLEAR. There are no more attacks of MS during the nine months of pregnancy than would be expected in women with MS who were not pregnant for nine months. Pregnancy does not appear to increase the incidence of attacks of MS; in fact, some data suggest that disease activity decreases during this period. However, there is an increased number of episodes of symptoms or attacks in the six months following delivery than would be expected in a six-month period. Those episodes should be treated and managed like any other episode of MS.

Two other aspects of pregnancy and child-rearing must be considered. First, there is a small but real genetic risk for MS in a family, in the range of 2–5 percent. This is greater than the risk in the normal population, but it is clearly very low. More significantly, raising a child is a lifelong responsibility, and people with MS must recognize that their health during the time that they will need to carry out this responsibility may be uncertain. One cannot predict health status in ten years, for example. This is probably the major factor that determines what people decide about raising a family. Recognizing the risks and problems, each couple must determine for themselves the very personal decision about having a child.

Will MS Affect My Sex Life?

BECAUSE MS AFFECTS THE CENTRAL NERVOUS SYSTEM AND THE NERVES THAT control various functions in the body, the complex and sensitive control system for sexual function can also be affected. Early in the disease there may be no physical effect on sexual function, but the enjoyment of sex may be affected by your emotional state. Worries, depression, or altered feelings about yourself can affect your relationship with others and the normal emotions associated with sexuality. Thus, sexual function may be affected by psychological factors, and this possibility needs to be considered. More often there is a physiological basis for the difficulties, which are often seen in conjunction with bladder and bowel symptoms. For men, the most common problem is achieving or maintaining an erection, which can be helped by medication. Women may experience decreased vaginal lubrication, which can be accommodated by synthetic lubricating products, such as Astroglide®.

What About Driving?

DRIVING IS ONLY A PROBLEM WHEN SYMPTOMS OR LIMITATIONS MAKE IT risky or unacceptably difficult. Vertigo, double vision, or a temporary loss of vision would not permit you to drive safely while you are experiencing them. Problems with leg weakness or incoordination would limit rapid and accurate use of brake and accelerator pedals and would make driving unsafe. It may be possible to return to driving when symptoms improve, but it is wise to depend on the assessment of your physician when there is any question about this. There are official driving testing centers, usually located at rehabilitation facilities, that can assess whether a person can drive safely. When a problem is more long-standing and renders driving unsafe, it may be possible to adapt the controls on the vehicle to allow a person to drive. The most common adaptation is alteration of the controls so that they are operated manually.

Although a person may be anxious to continue driving and willing to take some chances, feeling that they are "all right to drive," greater consideration must be given to others who may be at risk, including passengers or children in the street.

Should I Move?

SOME PEOPLE READ THAT THE INCIDENCE OF MS VARIES IN DIFFERENT PARTS of the world, that it is more common in temperate climates and rare in very hot climates, such as near the equator. They ask if it would be helpful if they moved to a hot climate; the answer is no. In fact they might find the heat a problem because it tends to make people with MS feel worse. We also believe that the geographic patterns probably have other explanations, such as the distribution in the world of people who have the genetic characteristic that might predispose to MS.

Will I Be Different?

IT IS NATURAL TO WONDER HOW MS WILL CHANGE YOU. YOUNG PEOPLE see themselves as healthy and do not visualize themselves with a serious disease. When you are given a diagnosis of a medical condition, it is natural to begin to think of yourself differently, and you may have to readjust your self-concept. You are still you, but it requires you to see that a different element has entered your life. Many things change as you go through life, some good, some not so good. What is necessary is a positive approach to challenges and determination to move ahead.

What About Other Questions I May Have?

WE COULD NOT POSSIBLY ANTICIPATE ALL THE QUESTIONS YOU MAY HAVE about what to do and not to do but we have tried to anticipate the most common ones. You will have many more questions, and they should be asked of your physician, other health care professionals, or staff at the MS Society. It is always better to ask a question, even if you are uncertain about exactly how to ask it or if you think it sounds "silly." It is better to ask a question than to wonder or worry in silence.

We recommend the book *Multiple Sclerosis: The Questions You Have—The Answers You Need* as a more detailed guide to many of your questions (see "Additional Reading").

5

Coping with Multiple Sclerosis

BEING DIAGNOSED WITH MULTIPLE SCLEROSIS CAN CREATE
turmoil in every area of a person's life. In some ways, life
will never be quite the same again. Even in the absence of
impairment, the worry—or efforts to camouflage worry—is
always there. The diagnosis often precipitates a roller
coaster ride of emotions, including fear, optimism, despair,
and hope. The time following diagnosis can be challenging
and confusing. This chapter is intended to give some order
to the emotional turmoil and help you think about ways to
ease the distress and continue with your life.

The Crisis of Diagnosis

People have a variety of reactions to hearing the diagnosis of MS for the
first time. Some people experience a combination of fear and panic when
first confronted with the news. These feelings may quickly be replaced
by denial, a refusal to believe that this could possibly be happening.
"There must be some mistake!" is an almost universal reaction to the diagnosis, often followed quickly by feelings of anger and resentment. Lisa's
story provides an example of some of these feelings. When asked about
her initial experience with MS and the diagnosis, she replied:

I was having a multitude of symptoms that I didn't understand, such as tingling and numbness in my hands and arms and legs. I was having trouble feeling the ground when I was walking. I couldn't see very well out of my left eye—it was almost like looking through an oily film. A whole bunch of odd things were happening that I didn't understand. . . . When I finally got the diagnosis, I was really scared. I didn't know what MS was or what would happen to me. I was afraid of the whole thing.

Later I was angry—very angry. Then I decided there was no way I could really have this disease. In fact, I was second-guessing the doctors—going from one to another asking what was wrong with me. All I could think of was that can in the grocery store that you throw your loose change into—you know, the one with the picture of someone in a wheelchair. It was probably a good year before I even started to accept the fact that I have MS. There was no way I could have it—I'm too active and I do so many things. And I can't stop doing them.

The diagnosis actually brings a sense of relief for some people, especially those who were beginning to wonder if they were "going crazy" or if the symptoms were "all in their head." These fears are sometimes reinforced by physicians who, in the absence of clear physical abnormalities, believe that emotional problems may be causing imaginary or exaggerated symptoms. A small study by Loveland (National MS Society, Health Services Research Report, 1993) found that women presenting with early symptoms of MS were significantly more likely than men to get this type of response from their doctors, and that men's descriptions of physical symptoms were generally given more credence by their physicians.

Relief is also experienced by those who imagined a more distressing, or perhaps fatal, explanation for their symptoms, such as cancer. Freed from the fears of a malignant tumor, they feel confident that the symptoms they are experiencing can be successfully managed.

Jim, who was diagnosed with MS in 1988 after a long and frustrating search for some answers, spoke about fear and relief at finally learning his diagnosis:

It took me eight years to get a diagnosis. I was scared to death when I heard "MS." I didn't even know what MS was. But I was also relieved. When you're used to not having a label for all the strange things that are going on and suddenly the problem is identified for you, that alone is a relief—all this finally has a name.

Regardless of the initial emotional response, the diagnosis of multiple sclerosis creates a crisis for the individual and the entire family. The person who has been diagnosed may experience a sense of isolation, despite efforts of family members to offer support. Lisa mentioned this experience:

> Even though people wanted to help, I was the one who had to learn to live with it and had to learn what I needed to do to live with it. You have to make your choice of how you're going to live your life. You have to do it because it's your disease and nobody can do it for you or make it go away.

Family members are also immersed in their own concerns about the future and the impact that MS will have on their lives. The positive aspect of this type of crisis is that it provides an opportunity to assess future plans and a powerful motivation to take actions that support those plans. There is an opportunity to affirm the values and strengths of the individual and the family and all the good things that remain intact in spite of MS. In order to go forward, it is important to know that you can successfully move through the difficult emotions and continue to pursue your goals and dreams.

The Adjustment Process

The initial variable reactions to the diagnosis of MS inevitably give way to a feeling of deep sadness. This is related to the addition of a serious chronic illness to one's identity and self-image. Chronic illness forces each person to confront the frailty and vulnerability of the human condition in a personal and immediate way. One also faces the painful reality of society's negative attitudes about disease and disability. This process involves grieving for one's former self-image and integrating the realities of MS into one's identity. Sadness, anger at the disease, and self-absorption are experienced during this time.

Grieving is necessary for a person to move forward, just as it is following the loss of a loved one. Unlike the grieving we associate with death, however, the grieving process in chronic illness tends to ebb and flow with the symptoms and physical changes that occur over time. Grief may be postponed but it can never be totally avoided. Sometimes these feelings may be channeled inappropriately, such as anger at one's spouse or children or at health professionals who cannot cure the illness. It is important for everyone involved to understand this grieving process and to communicate their care and support.

The period of intense grieving may last from a few weeks to several months, with gradually diminishing intensity. As it subsides, at least for the time being, one can begin again to focus on and enjoy special relationships and daily activities. Ideally, there is a gradual acknowledgment of the permanence of MS in one's life, while maintaining a sense of continuity between the past and the future as well as a commitment to maximizing quality of life.

Depressive feelings are to be expected as part of the initial grieving process or in response to subsequent changes or losses imposed by the illness. Over the course of the disease, however, individuals with multiple sclerosis seem to be at greater than average risk for depression. They need to be able to recognize when some kind of treatment intervention would be beneficial. Symptoms of significant depression include ongoing and pervasive sadness, loss of interest in or enjoyment of important activities and relationships, feelings of hopelessness and despair, sometimes including suicidal feelings or thoughts, and changes in sleeping and eating patterns. Intervention is recommended if any of these symptoms continue for an extended period of time or seem to be worsening. It is important to realize that relief from depression is readily available. Counseling and/or antidepressant medication are successful in relieving its symptoms. Seeking help for this problem demonstrates an understanding of its significance, not personal weakness or deficiency. Jim comments on his experience with depression:

> I was pretty depressed, so I went to see a psychologist. She was connected with a rehabilitation facility, so her primary interest was working with people who are chronically ill or disabled to help them find comfortable ways of living and thinking about themselves. It was a perfect match because that's just what I needed at that point.

A hallmark of MS that must be addressed as part of the adjustment process in its "unpredictability." When several focus groups were held by the National MS Society to identify what aspects of the disease people found most troubling and challenging, the resounding answer was the unpredictability of the disease course and the uncertainties related to future ability/disability. What symptoms and impairments might occur, when would new symptoms appear, when would they go away, or would they go away? Amy, who was diagnosed eight years ago, addressed this issue:

I think not knowing what will happen is the hardest thing for people when they're diagnosed with MS. They totally freak out and wonder "what's this disease going to do to me?" They have to realize that what happens to someone else is not necessarily going to happen to them. And if it does, well, you will have to deal with it.

Flexibility is a key element in living with the unpredictability of MS. Goals need to be assessed and revised, with a "plan for the worst, hope for the best" outlook. A college student named Leslie was pursuing a career in horticulture, which necessitated spending a fair amount of time in greenhouses. Her early symptoms included heat sensitivity, with temporary blurred vision and extreme fatigue when she was exposed to warm temperatures. Although this problem remitted, any future recurrence would have prevented Leslie from performing her job. After careful thought, she switched to teaching, an occupation in which heat sensitivity or most other possible MS symptoms would not prevent her from pursuing her career. Similarly, the purchase of a new home should involve consideration of issues of mobility and accessibility. Many people with MS are not significantly bothered by problems with walking. However, since mobility impairment is a problem at some point for a fair number of people with MS, it is simply good planning to consider this possibility when choosing a home, even while being reasonably optimistic that serious walking disturbances will not occur.

Coping Strategies

Coping strategies reflect an individual's personality and usual style of interfacing with people and events. By adulthood, strategies have been selected and refined though an unconscious process; most of us do not consciously choose and evaluate our coping mechanisms. However, it becomes important to look at those coping styles critically, so that they can be boosted when necessary and modified or discarded when they are counterproductive. The following are examples of two types of strategies.

Denial is ignoring or minimizing the seriousness of the situation. We all engage in denial about the moment-to-moment possibility of accidental death. Denial is useful in the early stages of adapting to MS because it enables people to deal with the immediate symptoms they are experiencing without having to contemplate all the possible problems that may occur in the future. Denial is *not* useful if these potential problems are ignored when making important life planning decisions such as purchasing disability insurance, buying a home or an automobile, or making career decisions. Denial can also interfere with obtaining optimal health care. Yes, a bladder infection may indicate underlying MS pathology and should be evaluated in light of that possibility. The numbness and tingling in your fingers may not be carpal tunnel syndrome, common now with almost universal computer use. Acknowledgment of your symptoms and paying proper attention to them will ensure that the physicians involved in your health care will provide you with the treatments you need and will not perform operations (e.g., for carpal tunnel syndrome or herniated disks) or prescribe treatments that are unnecessary or even harmful.

Intellectualization is focusing on available factual information to the exclusion of feelings and other psychological issues. A certain amount of intellectualization makes it possible for people to learn about the disease, assess its impact on their daily lives, and make use of their problem-solving abilities to meet the challenges imposed by MS. Intellectualization becomes excessive when it consumes enormous amounts of energy; some people expend so much effort collecting and analyzing information that they have little or no energy left to deal with their emotional reactions to the disease or with the feelings and reactions of those around them.

Looking at these two examples, the strengths and weaknesses inherent in some coping strategies can be seen. Denial is useful in allowing a person to get on with his or her life, but detrimental if it interferes with obtaining optimal treatment or with life planning issues. Intellectualization is useful in obtaining essential information, but harmful when it is used as a means of blocking feelings about the disease that should be expressed. The blocking of emotional awareness and expression can interfere with long-range coping efforts.

Interpersonal difficulties can arise when two people who live together and must cope with MS have conflicting coping styles. A person who copes by talking through feelings and events or by reading all the literature on MS may encounter resistance and even anger from a partner who is trying desperately to maintain denial as a way of dealing with the disease. In some situations, counseling is useful to help a couple recognize each other's coping styles and provide mutual support.

Education About MS

While some individuals are more inclined than others to seek information about something that is stressful to them, one of the most effective things a person with MS or a family member can do to facilitate adjustment to MS is to learn about the disease—what to expect and what can be done to relieve physical symptoms and promote psychological health. People with MS have indicated in National MS Society surveys that information about the disease and its effects is their most important need. Education about MS is available through a number of sources, primarily MS health care providers and the U.S. and Canadian MS Societies (see Chapter 9).

Keep in mind, however, that adults can choose to learn in a variety of ways, and may choose to do so in different settings or at different times. For some, devouring every available piece of written material is the most desirable strategy. These individuals compare different sources of information, analyzing and sorting varied opinions, to create a personal perspective. The result is a sense of "ownership" over the information and its gradual integration into personal philosophy and decisions about day-to-day activities. Other people prefer a group setting that provides opportunities for the immediate testing of new ideas and feedback from peers and/or professionals. Such group educational programs are widely available through the U.S. and Canadian MS Societies. Some chapters in the United States also have a mail program, called "Knowledge Is Power," for people who have been recently diagnosed with MS. The program consists of a series of modules on topics of interest sent on a predetermined schedule to people who request this service.

Another component of the educational process relates to reports of possible treatments or "the cure" for MS. Given the variability and unpredictability of the illness over time, it is not surprising that diverse therapies have been heralded as having a significant impact on MS. When symptoms remit—as they frequently do quite naturally over the course of the disease—whatever treatment or activity is being used at the time is given credit for the improvement. Since dramatic improvement and long periods of remission are common occurrences in MS, even without any therapy, it is important to be prudently skeptical when evaluating therapies that claim to benefit people with MS. Only those treatments that have been evaluated for safety and efficacy in carefully designed and controlled scientific studies should be seriously considered.

Choice of Health Care Providers

The choice of health care providers is a critical decision relative to long-term management issues. People with MS generally have a normal life expectancy, and management of the disease is a lifelong process. The physician who manages the symptoms and disease course will interact with the other physicians involved in your health care, such as your internist, gynecologist/obstetrician, cardiologist, or any other medical specialist whose services you might require during your lifetime. Members of your chosen health care team will also provide you on an ongoing basis with information that you will need to make important life decisions relating, for example, to job choices, family planning, or the selection of an MS treatment option. Choose your health care providers carefully. Investigate your physician's board certification (neurology, physiatry, family practice, or internal medicine), experience with MS, hospital or medical center affiliation, and reputation in the community. The local chapter (United States) or division (Canada) of the MS Society can suggest several physicians in any given community who have experience in the management of MS, as well as MS specialists in certain geographic locations.

Support Networks

Family and friends provide the major support for the person who has MS. Their caring and concern are vital, especially during the difficult times following diagnosis or when a flare-up of symptoms occurs. A "sorting out" of friends and relatives may be necessary, since not all people with a close relationship are able to be supportive in the same way. One person may be comfortable listening to concerns and providing emotional support, while another may find it easier to assist with more concrete activities, such as a ride to the doctor's office. Another friend or relative may be a great problem-solver, helpful in finding solutions or identifying resources in troublesome situations. At the same time, a person's ability to help should not be too narrowly or rigidly determined, especially without discussing it with him or her. It is important for all those who provide support to know how important their contributions are to the person with MS.

People with MS may find it especially helpful to talk with other people who have the disease. This interaction helps to demonstrate that people with MS do indeed continue productive and satisfying lives despite the intrusion of the disease. A physician or other health care provider may be able to provide the name and phone number of someone who is willing, even eager, to talk about his or her personal experiences with MS.

Many chapters of the National MS Society have "peer counseling" programs that train selected individuals with MS to be helpful to people who have questions about the disease. They are available to answer questions, discuss issues, and relate their personal MS successes and failures. In some areas, the peer counselor is available for a telephone conversation; in others, the counselor may also be available at local MS center (medical) sessions. Amy commented on her experience with a peer counselor:

> *Having that one-on-one interaction, having someone to talk to who understands, who has gone through similar experiences—that was really important to me. She was a source of strength and kept helping my self-image to stay in shape.*

Some people find a group setting most helpful because they can benefit from the experiences of a number of people with MS. Group members also feel good about the group interaction and support, which is much like a family support network. In an MS support group, MS temporarily feels "normal," since it is the common experience of all members. This normalization of MS is extremely supportive of the overall adjustment process. Instead of feeling isolated, the person in a support (often self-help) group sees MS as one component of a full and diverse life, which can be managed with an understanding of the disease, support of family, friends, health professionals, and peers with MS.

Disclosure

Disclosure about one's illness—whether to family members and friends, new acquaintances, or employers and colleagues—is a significant issue for most people living with MS. Many people are uncertain how much information they want or need to disclose, especially because there is often no visible impairment, and some of the symptoms caused by the illness can easily be attributed to a less serious cause. Considerations about disclosure at the workplace are discussed in Chapter 9.

The first and most important group or people to consider are your family members. They are the easiest to make recommendations about, but sometimes the most difficult group to tell. Close family members need to know about your MS—what to expect and what they can do to help. In general, parents, siblings, and other close adult relatives should be told calmly and directly about the diagnosis. They need to begin learning what MS is and what is known about the person's prognosis and limitations.

Children should also be told about the diagnosis. Even very young children are aware when something is wrong and imagine the worst possible scenario. They need to be given some concrete information about the disease that they can relate to and understand, e.g., that Mommy will be extra tired sometimes, may have trouble walking, or will need to hurry to the toilet. They also need to be reassured that Mommy is not going to die and that she will be able to take of them. Children need to know that although the parent may not be able to be as physically active as before, the family will work together to solve any problems that arise. Parents should also explain that no one can "catch" MS the way a cold can be caught from another person, that the children did not cause the MS, and that they have no control over making it better or worse. Parents tend to underestimate the impact of MS on their children; they are at least as affected by their parents' emotional state and the emotional climate within the household as they are by any physical limitations imposed by illness.

What to tell friends and acquaintances may need to be determined on a case-by-case basis. How much you choose to tell will depend very much on the relationship you have with another person. Informing your friends will allow them to provide the emotional support you need and will also relieve you of energy-consuming efforts to conceal the problem.

Disclosure is also an issue for people who are dating. When is the best time to tell, and how much should be revealed? As with other questions about MS, no single answer suits every individual or situation. In general, you have no obligation to talk about your MS prior to extending or accepting an invitation for a date. Nor should you feel any need to discuss MS before you have decided whether you like a person. Once you have decided that a relationship is worth pursuing, the following guidelines may be helpful:

- remember that secrets and half-truths do not make a firm foundation for a healthy relationship;
- think about when you would like to know important health-related information about the other person;

- keep in mind that revealing your MS may become increasingly difficult as your investment in the relationship increases.

Wellness Orientation

In contrast to a disease orientation, which focuses on minimizing the impact of the chronic disease on all aspects of your life, a wellness approach looks at achieving the positive state of maximal health despite the presence of a chronic illness. Jones and Kilpatrick, in the *Families in Society Journal* (May 1996), propose a definition of wellness as the state of harmony, energy, positive productivity, and well-being in an individual's mind, body, emotions, and spirit. This model encompasses interpersonal relationships as well as relationships with the environment, the community, and society in general. The wellness orientation is comprehensive in its promotion of mind-body unity within the individual, as well as integration of the individual within the community and society as a whole.

A practical example of a wellness orientation is the exploration of aerobic and general conditioning exercises, which go beyond traditional physical therapy designed primarily to address disease-imposed impairments. Nutritional programs designed for general health, e.g., the prevention of heart disease and certain forms of cancer, go beyond traditional dietary measures that target specific MS-related problems such as constipation and urinary infections.

Practices such as yoga, meditation, and Tai Chi also fall within the wellness concept and are sometimes categorized as "complementary therapies" that work along with, rather than against or in place of, traditional medical therapy. The term *complementary therapy* is new and not clearly defined, with the result that certain non-medical therapies are considered unproven, speculative, or even dangerous by the medical community. However, there is growing support by medical professionals for a wellness orientation, as well as for selected aspects of complementary therapies. It is hoped that this shift in attitude will lead to more controlled studies of the risks and benefits of some of these therapies. Lisa again comments on her experiences, focusing on wellness behaviors:

I learned to watch fats and learned more about what I should eat. Now when I finish school I usually go straight to the swimming pool and exercise for thirty to forty minutes.

In following a wellness approach, it is important to remember that one cannot directly impact the disease process through health-promoting behaviors. People need to recognize that their control over MS is limited and that the disease may become active in spite of the health practices they have initiated. People should feel good about the wellness activities they pursue in order to enhance their general health and well-being, but they should not feel guilty or blame themselves if and when a relapse occurs. Although a wellness approach cannot control the unpredictable nature of MS, it can enable people to improve their health and devise creative ways to continue activities that are satisfying and enjoyable.

Similarly, people often believe that they can control their MS if they simply try hard enough to "fight" it. Those who engage in this kind of thinking tend to experience a sense of failure when the disease worsens. Assuming this kind of personal responsibility for disease progression is both harmful and self-defeating. Your energy, emotional and otherwise, is better channeled into pursuing wellness, always recognizing that the goal is overall improvement in general health rather than control of the disease process.

Individuals who struggle to control their MS sometimes feel that they are losing the battle or "giving up" if they begin to use an assistive device. These devices actually *extend* your abilities by conserving energy, promoting safety, and reducing effort. For example, those who fatigue easily or struggle to be ambulatory with a cane or crutches will find that their activities become severely limited. All their energy is used simply to get from one place to another, leaving little or none to do or enjoy whatever activity had been planned. Struggling to get to the supermarket may mean that there is no energy left to shop upon arrival. People with MS need to use whatever techniques, tools, or devices are available to maximize and extend their activities and opportunities. Someone who is comfortable walking for short distances may choose to use a motorized scooter on a trip to an amusement park, shopping mall, or museum. A worker in a large office who normally uses a cane might also choose to use a scooter to conserve energy and enhance productivity. The effective use of assistive devices is an important extension of the wellness philosophy. These tools should be seen as a means of maintaining a full, productive, and enjoyable life rather than as a symbol of defeat.

Parting Thoughts

Lisa relates her personal philosophy:

> *If I had never had MS, I would never have traveled the way I did. I took a year off after I was diagnosed and traveled all around Europe. I decided I was going to do things while I could because I didn't know when something might be taken away from me. And I think one thing I've learned from MS is to do things while I can. It's a lesson for everyone. We should all live each day to the fullest, because we never know when something might happen to take it away.*

Jim relates what gets him through:

> *I would say that I have a lot of support from my family and friends. That probably helped me through. I had quite a few conversations, talks, heart-to-heart discussions with different people and that helped me quite a bit. Also, I'm somewhat religious and that helped.*

A religious or spiritual orientation has been linked with successful coping in a number of studies. It seems that religion helps some people find meaning in their illness or at least put it into a meaningful context. Amy also refers to spirituality, as well as her own personal characteristics, as a support:

> *Since I grew up in a single parent household, I always had to draw on my own resources. So I worked real hard on that—and on my own sense of spirituality. I just had to—I've always depended on myself. I've always demanded a lot from myself and I guess I just drew it from within.*

Amy refers to a key aspect of the coping process—a person's inner strengths. With an adult-onset disease, coping strategies have already been tested in other areas, creating a base on which to build. These strengths surface as the sense of crisis recedes. Amy has more advice for dealing with MS and with life in general.

> *Another thing is to laugh—to have a sense of humor. Don't take things so seriously. If you don't have a sense of humor, it's all for naught, you know. Life is too short. It can just really drag you down if you let it— you can't let that happen. Just try to take things one day at a time. One day at a time and "slow is fast enough," you don't really have to be in that much of a hurry. Take your time and take it easy and don't be afraid to ask for help.*

6

Employment Issues and Multiple Sclerosis

MOST ADULTS SPEND THE MAJORITY OF THEIR WAKING HOURS at work and have a serious personal investment in and commitment to employment-related activities. A person's self-image and identity are often drawn from his or her occupation or professional status. One of the first questions asked when getting to know someone is "What kind of work do you do?" From a practical perspective, income generated as wages is necessary to purchase goods and services to maintain a particular lifestyle for the individual and his or her family. Work without direct financial remuneration, such as parenting, homemaking, and volunteer activities, also contribute to self-definition, but usually without the lifestyle consequences. These activities, however, will also have financial impact if they must be replaced by the work of salaried personnel. Given these factors, it is not surprising that anything that potentially threatens the ability to continue employment or other productive and rewarding activity generates concern and anxiety. A diagnosis of multiple sclerosis certainly presents this kind of distressing situation.

The good news is that most people who discover that they have MS can and should continue working, usually in their current capacity. Symptoms experienced during a flare-up of the disease may or may not interfere with ability to function at work, but in most cases the prior activity level can be continued. Even when an exacerbation precludes usual work activities, these episodes only occur on the average of one to two per year in the relapsing-remitting form of the disease. Progressive MS may require some changes, but disease limitations appear at a slow enough pace to allow for necessary modifications.

A person with a recent diagnosis of multiple sclerosis may not quickly or easily arrive at a comfort level with the disease and work-related issues. The emotions surrounding this unpleasant news are likely to engulf work areas as well as almost all aspects of a person's day-to-day life. Even when most physical symptoms have cleared, unpleasant and troubling invisible symptoms may remain. Problems such as fatigue, numbness, or pain can increase anxiety and interfere with actual job activities. Symptoms such as urinary urgency and frequency may cause embarrassment. Impaired balance can be socially distressing because of the association with drinking an excessive amount of alcohol.

These factors are mentioned to highlight the emotional turmoil a person newly diagnosed with MS may experience. This is not the frame of mind to have when making critical decisions about work. TAKE YOUR TIME. Be sure that you have accurate and sufficient information on which to base a decision, and that you are emotionally prepared to look objectively at the entire situation—know all your options and their ramifications. Speak with others who have successfully managed MS and/or with a counselor who is experienced in helping people with MS think through the important issues related to employment.

With this background in mind, the following critical points must be emphasized:

- employment and other productive activities must not be abandoned unnecessarily because of fear and/or misinformation;
- help is available to assist with work-related decisions and to implement the steps necessary to keep working.

Myths About Multiple Sclerosis

There are a number of myths or false beliefs that make adjustment to multiple sclerosis problematic. These misconceptions are held not only by a segment of the general public, but also by an alarming number of health professionals who do not have extensive experience with MS and/or are unfamiliar with the MS professional literature. Some of these myths have a direct impact on the work experience.

- *Stress.* At various points in the history of MS, stress was thought to worsen the disease and escalate the disease process. Scientific studies have looked at this issue in detail, and results have failed to support the role of stress in either the onset or the progression of MS. Advice to quit working, get help to care for children, and curtail volunteer activities is misguided if it is based only on the *diagnosis* of MS. Specific symptoms may have an impact, but they need to be evaluated individually and carefully since problems may be self-limited or responsive to symptomatic therapy.
- *Activity.* It was formerly believed that physical activity was detrimental to people with MS. The directive was to "take it easy," stop all physical exercise, and rest as much as possible. Bed rest was the primary recommendation for this erratic and unpredictable disease. The major public figure to challenge this notion was Olympic ski medalist Jimmie Heuga, who could not accept a life of inactivity. We now know that Jimmie was right, that activity and exercise are actually beneficial to the well-being of people with MS. It follows that work-related activity should not be curtailed unless dictated by specific, long-standing symptoms that have not responded to therapy.
- *Incapacitation.* Prior to MS being recognized in early stages and mild cases, the common belief was that it would inevitably, and usually quickly, lead to serious disability interfering with the ability to perform daily activities, including employment. It is now known that this is not true and that most people with MS can remain active and involved.

Disclosure

The decision to communicate—or not to communicate—the diagnosis of MS at the workplace is complex and important, and deserves careful consideration. Disclosure when interviewing for a new job poses different issues from disclosure when one already holds an established position.

It is important to be aware of both legal and practical considerations, whether seeking a new job or maintaining a current one. In the United States, people with disabilities are protected by the Americans with Disabilities Act (ADA), which became law in 1990. The definition of "disability" is complex, but it clearly encompasses MS regardless of whether symptoms are present or not. This is due to the possible *perception* of a disability. A diagnosis of MS carries such a possible preconception, since an employer could potentially discriminate based on the association of MS with disability. The ADA prohibits employers from asking about or considering a diagnosis or general limitations in hiring and promotion decisions, and only allows questions about ability to perform key components of the job. The job applicant or employee need only be armed with information related to key job components, and need not be concerned about responses to disease or disability-related questions, as long as the capacity to perform the job is not compromised. It is important to think about the essential or key elements of your current or prospective job, since non-essential functions may legally be delegated to or traded with other employees.

In a similar manner, Canadians are protected by the Employment Equity Act (Bill C-64) passed in 1995, which replaces the previous Employment Equity Act (EE Act). This legislation eliminates employment barriers experienced by women, Aboriginals, and visible minorities, as well as people with disabilities. In a news release at the time of passage, Art Eggleton, President of the Treasury Board, described how employment equity was being advanced while the talents and expertise of all Canadians were being promoted. Among the areas of concern that prompted this most recent employment antidiscrimination legislation was the severe underrepresentation in the workplace of people with disabilities. Both the private and public sectors are covered by Bill C-64. The Act makes use of the Canadian Human Rights Tribunal (to be named the Employment Equity Review Tribunal when hearing employment equity cases). It also confirms the mandate for Human Resources Development Canada to conduct research, provide labor market data, and administer programs to recognize outstanding achievement in employment equity. Both appeal procedures and enforcement measures are addressed.

Apart from legal considerations, people with MS have concerns about health insurance, life insurance, and disability insurance. The prospective or current employee needs to explore policies relative to diagnosis of a chronic disease or occurrence of disability. "Preexisting condition" clauses must be carefully investigated, as well as "caps" (lifetime limits on expenditures for a particular condition or for an individual's total medical expenses) and related categories that potentially limit the availability of medical and health services because of MS or another chronic condition. These factors may or may not be disclosure-related, depending on prior documentation of diagnosis and extent of information required for ongoing insurance coverage.

The non-insurance, non-legal aspects of working with MS are often more difficult to assess and address. Such considerations include anticipated employer and fellow employee support or lack of support, possible growth freeze if limitations are imagined by the employer, and personal emotional investment in efforts to acknowledge or deny issues related to MS. Colleagues, including supervisors, often rally to support a fellow worker with a health problem and pull in resources such as "matching gifts" or volunteer incentives. Disclosure allows the individual to relieve the stress of covering up real needs and concerns and to mobilize team spirit and support. It is also necessary to disclose necessary accommodations. The employer is required to make arrangements to help the employee perform "essential job functions." These accommodations must be "reasonable" in that they must be affordable and must not impose undue hardship on the employer.

There are also compelling reasons not to disclose: subtle or not so subtle pressure to resign, to accept lesser job responsibilities, or not to apply for promotion or expanded responsibilities. People have reported a "dead end" feeling, where the supervisor has clearly communicated lack of support for further advancement.

Resources

This information is not likely to be needed now, and may never be needed. However, awareness is critical at the time of diagnosis so that appropriate assistance can be obtained at the first sign of difficulty and larger problems can be avoided altogether. Modest effort early on can prevent serious situations later and can support smooth career development.

Literature is available from the National Multiple Sclerosis Society in the United States (800-FIGHT-MS) and the Multiple Sclerosis Society of Canada (416-922-6065). Two booklets are particularly helpful:

ADA and People with MS (Cooper and Law, 1994), which gives details about your protection under the law in an easy-to-read style, and *The Win-Win Approach to Reasonable Accommodations* (Rumrill, 1995), which deals with the employer-employee relationship when an "accommodation" is needed. An accommodation may involve a change in scheduling, a parking space closer to the building entrance, or an office closer to the bathroom. Occasionally equipment or a structural change such as a ramp may be needed. This is less often the case, but is usually accomplished with minimal effort and cost when dealt with directly when the need is first identified.

Most National MS Society chapters have periodic educational programs that target people recently diagnosed with MS and their families, and include issues relative to employment. Each state has a vocational rehabilitation office; the number can be obtained through the telephone directory or information assistance. Look in the blue government pages of the telephone book under "State Government," then look under one of the following headings:

Department of Vocational Rehabilitation
Department of Rehabilitation
Department of Human Services
Department of Social Services
Department of Social & Rehabilitation Services.

Some important resources include:

- *Technical Assistance Centers*

- *National Institute on Disability & Rehabilitation Research*
  1-800-949-4232
  202-205-9151(voice), 202-205-9136 (TDD)

- *Equal Employment Opportunities Commission (EEOC) District/ National Office*
  800-669-4000 to speak with an agent
  800-669-EEOC (3362) for written information
  800-669-6820 (TDD)

- *Architectural & Transportation Barriers Compliance Board*
  800-USA-ABLE (872-2253)
  (202) 272-5434 (voice)

Other resources in Canada include:

- *Barrier-Free Design Centre (at Access Place Canada)*
  College Park
  444 Yonge Street
  Toronto, Ontario M5B 2H4
  416-977-5010

- *Canadian Council on Rehabilitation and Work*
  410-167 Lombard Avenue
  Winnipeg, Manitoba R3B OT6
  204-942-44862

- *Canadian Institute for Barrier-Free Design Faculty of Architecture*
  University of Manitoba
  Winnipeg, Manitoba R3T 2N2
  204-474-6450

- *Canadian Rehabilitation Council for the Disabled*
  45 Sheppard Avenue East, Suite 801
  Toronto, Ontario M2N 5W9
  416-250-7490 (voice and TDD for hearing impaired)

- *Jancana—The Job Accommodation Network in Canada*
  c/o 410-167 Lombard Avenue
  Winnipeg, Manitoba R3B OT6
  800-526-2262

7

Research in Multiple Sclerosis: The Search for Answers

RESEARCH INTO MS BEGAN IN THE MID-1800S AS SIMPLE descriptive studies that examined the symptoms of the disease and its effect on nervous system tissue. MS research has evolved into a specialty area of basic and clinical research that incorporates virtually every discipline of modern biotechnology, ranging from the most esoteric laboratory techniques to studies of population, socioeconomics, and psychology, and to the testing new therapies for their safety and efficacy.

Scientific research is in itself a specialized discipline. Scientists are trained not only in their area of specialty research but also in the discipline of scientific inquiry. Simple "observation" is a form of scientific inquiry that is most useful in initial studies. In its most rigorous form, scientific research involves the testing of specific theories or hypotheses, using controlled laboratory or clinical techniques that have the greatest likelihood of providing meaningful answers. A *hypothesis* is a tentative assumption that a scientist seeks to prove or disprove in the course of investigation, using state-of-the-art technology to get complete answers.

Most modern MS research is related to the four major hypotheses surrounding the disease and its cause (see Chapter 2): that it is an autoimmune disease; that it occurs in genetically susceptible individuals; that it is triggered by some infectious or environmental factor (perhaps a virus infection); and that it results in inflammation and loss of the white matter of the brain and spinal cord, bringing neurologic symptoms and the associated socioeconomic problems long recognized to be aspects of MS.

Research in Immunology

While MS is recognized as a disease of the brain and spinal cord of the central nervous system (CNS), it is widely believed that the characteristic neurologic signs and symptoms of MS are caused by an immune system disorder that causes damage to CNS tissue and disrupts the normal activity of the CNS that allows movement, sensory perception, thinking and emotional functioning.

The immune system is a highly complex organ of the body that includes lymphocytes (T cells), antibodies, a host of regulatory substances that circulate in the blood called cytokines, and many other key players. Normal immune function protects the body from injury and disease caused by infectious agents—bacteria, viruses, parasites, and the like—by mounting an attack against the "invaders" and clearing them from the body. Our own body tissues are generally protected against attack by our immune system.

While there is some disagreement, most scientists working in the field of MS believe that the disease is caused by an abnormality in which a person's own immune system fails to distinguish foreign invaders— bacteria, viruses, parasites—from normal tissue in the body. As a consequence, the immune system attacks normal body tissue, resulting in inflammation and tissue damage that is often permanent. This "self-attack" of the immune system against body tissues is termed "autoimmunity." Autoimmunity, then, is considered to be the true root cause of MS, and as such is perhaps the largest area of research in MS worldwide. Understanding immune function in the disease will help pinpoint its cause and will result in innovate new therapies.

Immunologic research related to MS has progressed over a number of years from identifying immune cells in the nervous system, where they do not normally belong, to understanding how immune system components are regulated and become dysfunctional in autoimmune disease. We are now in a position to marshal this vital information about immune system function and dysfunction into the development of potential new therapies for MS.

Studies have been undertaken in healthy individuals to better understand normal immune system functioning, in individuals with MS to understand what goes wrong in the disease, and in individuals with other autoimmune diseases, such as rheumatoid arthritis and juvenile onset diabetes, to understand what they can tell us more generally about the immune system abnormality.

In addition to human studies, immunologic research in MS has been greatly aided by work on the laboratory animal model disease, experimental allergic encephalomyelitis (EAE), an autoimmune disease of the brain and spinal cord in laboratory rats, mice, guinea pigs, and primates that has many characteristics in common with MS. Studies of animal models for MS and related animal model diseases for other human autoimmune disorders have greatly facilitated our understanding of basic immune system function and what goes wrong in autoimmune diseases and are a practical, relatively rapid way to obtain answers to difficult questions.

Because MS involves the immune system, for several decades physicians have used strong drugs that suppress immune function by decreasing growth and proliferation of immune cells. Many experimental therapies tested for MS had global or widespread immunosuppressive effects, leaving a treated patient open to a variety of infections and complications, which made these therapies of questionable value. Pinpointing the scope of immune problems in the disease has long been a goal, with the belief that such information could lead to highly specific therapies aimed at those immune system components involved in the disease, leaving the rest of the immune system intact and functioning.

The search to understand the specific immune responses involved in MS has been an important focus of research in recent years. This includes exploring what makes an immune system that is normally directed against outside invaders become misdirected against normal body tissues; searching for the actual target of immune responses in the brain and spinal cord (the "antigen"); and determining the nature of T cells and antibodies that are primed to attack this target.

Another promising avenue of immunology research seeks to understand how and why immune system cells and antibodies move from the blood stream into the CNS. Work in this area is essential if we are to complete the picture of MS and develop treatments that prevent such "trafficking" and stop the disease in its tracks.

Not all hypotheses and studies are successful in MS research (or in any other branch of research). For instance, in the late 1980s, with considerable background information on immune responses in EAE in mice, scientists reported evidence that there were relatively few brain antigens—targets of the disease process—in myelin around nerve fibers. They also reported that they were able to identify T cells specific to those antigens and, they believed, to the MS disease process.

With this information, a number of scientists and pharmaceutical companies began to design specifically engineered antibodies (immune system proteins produced in the laboratory that have an ability to target and "neutralize" specific proteins) and synthetic peptides (parts of proteins) aimed at preventing immune system attack against the CNS. In the animal disease, EAE, disease could be prevented entirely and improvement was seen when disease was already present before treatment.

While such information generated enormous excitement and many hypotheses for treating MS in humans, the immune response against myelin in humans turned out to be much more complicated than in the laboratory animal model disease. There are clearly a number of myelin antigens involved in immune system responses in humans, and different people may have different antigen responses. Over time, there tends to be a shifting in immune responses so that the target of the immune response in myelin may change. This means that specific T cell treatments are not likely to be effective for a wide spectrum of patients with MS, and treatments effective at one time in the disease may not continue to be effective over time.

One consequence of these disappointments has been a focus in immunology research in MS on chemical messengers called cytokines. Cytokines are produced by immune and other cells that regulate immune system activity. Many scientists believe that they may be important "final pathways" involved in all immune responses, and that by manipulating cytokine activity it may not be necessary to understand specific immune cell responses in MS to combat the disease. Early studies showed that some cytokines make EAE or MS worse and others may make the diseases better. Interferons, which are one type of cytokine, are an example of this dichotomy: interferon beta has been shown to be beneficial for treating MS, while there is evidence that interferon gamma makes the disease worse. Work is underway to gain a better understanding of the cytokine "networks" that are involved in MS and to learn how to block "bad" cytokines and enhance the effects of "good" ones, all to the ultimate goal of providing safe and effective disease treatments.

An enormous amount has been learned about specific immune system responses in MS and even this "blind alley" has generated new concepts in autoimmunity and how autoimmune diseases may be regulated and controlled. Work progresses at a more rapid pace than ever before.

Genetic Research

Understanding genetic factors in MS is a relatively new and rapidly expanding field, resulting in vast amounts of new information. Basic population studies (still under way) tell us that there are specific groups of people in the world that may be protected from MS and others that may be more susceptible (see Chapter 2). Now genetic research has become highly "molecular" in nature, as scientists race to uncover genetic factors that underlie the disease and may help determine who is susceptible to developing MS.

The possibility of specific gene therapies is no longer the stuff of science fiction, even though its application to human disease is far from straightforward today. A more immediate consequence of such genetic work may be development of techniques to more readily determine susceptibility to MS in the general population and in families in which the disease already occurs. Genetic factors may even one day provide some clues to the prognosis for any individual with the disease.

An added boost to the belief that MS is autoimmune in nature comes from genetic studies. Immune function is under strict genetic control and the genes of people with MS that control immune function are in some ways apparently different from the immune system genes of healthy individuals. At their most basic level, genetic studies are helping us to know more about the immune nature of the disease, how much of the disease susceptibility may be related to genetic problems in immune system function, and how much of it may be related to other, non-immunologic factors, or even to environmental or infectious factors.

Major genetic breakthroughs have occurred in recent times, primarily relating to diseases such as Huntington's chorea and Duchenne muscular dystrophy, where a problem in a single, identifiable gene results in disease. Genetic studies in MS have shown that the genetic factors are far more complex, and that multiple genes are likely involved, perhaps even genes that would not be predicted based on the disease characteristics. By the mid-1990s three major "genetic screening" studies had begun in the United States, Canada, and Europe to search the complete set of human chromosomes (genome) for differences between those with MS and others (primarily unaffected family members) who do not have the disease. These complementary studies will do much to help us understand the complex genetic factors underlying MS.

By 1990 molecular genetic research had identified two types of immune system genes that might be involved in MS. The first are genes involved in helping the immune system determine which body tissues are its own ("self") and which substances are foreign—a bacteria or virus, or even a transplanted liver or kidney from a genetically different donor. This ability to distinguish between "self" and "foreign" allows the immune system to mount an effective response against foreign substances but not against "self" substances. Genes controlling this recognition process are called histocompatibility genes, human leukocyte antigens (HLA genes), or major histocompatibility genes (MHC genes).

The second important gene type that may be involved in MS controls structure and function of "receptors" on T cells of the immune system. Such receptors are essential in determining the target of immune responses. Some evidence, while still controversial, suggests that both HLA genes and T cell receptor genes in people with MS may be different from those in people without the disease.

Virus Research

Genes and the immune system are clearly involved with MS, but what event actually triggers the development of MS in people who are susceptible? That is where virus research has come in. Virus infections can cause diseases with characteristics similar to MS, and certain viral diseases in laboratory animals also result in myelin damage. There is also evidence that certain viral infections may set off acute exacerbations of MS in individuals who already have the disease.

For decades, researchers have hunted for a specific, identifiable virus related to MS. However, the search for "the" MS virus has proven unfruitful. Several dozen common and uncommon viruses have been postulated to be specifically related to MS, based either on epidemiology studies or the presence of higher levels of antibodies against a given virus in individuals with MS. In virtually every case, follow-up studies to demonstrate a relationship to MS have been unsuccessful; most have been determined to be due to inadequate experimental sampling or laboratory contamination. Nonetheless, there remains the possibility that specific infections may be related to MS, and virologists with a focus on this disease are at the forefront of ongoing searches.

Many believe it is likely that no specific virus or other infectious agent will be found to be related to MS. Rather, they are concentrating on research that explores how a susceptible person's immune system reacts to a variety of viral or other infections, or how immune function is tied to hormonal and other factors that might explain the initiation of the MS process. Studies in the mid-1990s, amplifying earlier studies on MS-like disease in animals, helped to explain how an immune system that has lost its ability to distinguish "self" from "non-self" tissue can be tricked by certain infectious agents into mounting an attack against a person's own myelin. This example of "mistaken identity" may explain much of the origin of MS and help to determine how the disease can be prevented from occurring in susceptible people.

Glial Cell Research

The symptoms of MS are due directly to inflammation and breakdown of myelin and cells that make myelin—called oligodendrocytes—in the brain and spinal cord of the CNS. The biology of oligodendrocytes and other such "glial" cells in the CNS is therefore a vital and expanding area of research. This includes study of how oligodendrocytes develop and form myelin in early stages of life, how they are affected by immune system responses, how the nervous system responds when myelin is lost, how scars are formed when myelin is lost, and what the potential is for myelin regeneration and recovery.

Basic biochemical studies of myelin using increasingly sophisticated techniques have closely analyzed the tissue in people with MS, and such studies are used to determine if there are any abnormalities in the myelin or oligodendrocytes that might make these tissues and cells vulnerable to immune system attack. Much traditional biochemistry has repeatedly demonstrated that myelin, or white matter, in individuals with MS is "normal," suggesting that the autoimmune attack in MS is truly a question of immune cells not recognizing normal, "self" tissue. By the mid-1990s, a new technology stemming from magnetic resonance imaging, called magnetic resonance spectroscopy, began to indicate that normal-appearing white matter in the brains of people with MS may have subtle abnormalities after all. It is not clear if this is directly related to a cause of the disease or whether it is an early, previously undetected result of the disease process. Such studies show not only the power of newer technologies but also the need to constantly reassess scientific beliefs and facts.

For many decades it was believed that myelin in the CNS could not be regenerated after it was damaged or lost in adults. This belief was shattered by the finding in the early 1980s that there was a degree of new myelin development in individuals whose brains showed extensive immune system damage and scarring due to MS. This myelin regeneration was weak, slow, and insufficient to overcome the devastation caused by the disease, but provided new hope that myelin could be repaired.

Primed by this relatively recent knowledge that damaged CNS oligodendrocytes can regenerate and form new myelin, many laboratories are focusing on ways to enhance myelin growth and development in animals and in humans. In most cases of MS, particularly early cases, myelin insulation around nerve fibers is damaged or lost, but the underlying nerve fibers that control functions are intact and would probably be able to function essentially normally if insulation were restored.

Some experimental approaches scientists are taking to meet this challenge include identifying the myelin-making cells in the nervous system that are capable of forming new tissue after immune system damage; using "growth factors" to stimulate more rapid and efficient myelin growth; modulating immune system functions that may be inhibiting myelin growth; and transplanting myelin-making cells from healthy "donors" to diseased or damaged nervous systems.

In the mid-1990s, these studies were largely limited to experimentation in laboratory animals with genetically deficient myelin or animals in which specific myelin lesions had been experimentally produced, but studies using certain immunoglobulins to suppress a theorized immunologic inhibition of myelin grown had begun in humans with MS. All of this work provides hope that myelin regrowth and functional recovery for individuals with MS may be possible in the future.

It is vital to recognize two key problems: as long as the immune system problems responsible for myelin destruction remain unchecked, any efforts at myelin regeneration will be sabotaged by the ongoing disease process; and, for some individuals with advanced MS, it is clear that there is damage not only to myelin but also to vital nerve fibers. Nerve fibers that are damaged are unlikely to be able to function again even if myelin insulation has been restored. Thus, research focusing on myelin regeneration must move hand-in-hand with efforts to stop the underlying immune system process.

Clinical Research

Clinical research directly involves individuals who have MS. It is aimed in a number of different directions. Studies in basic immunology, virology, and glial biology, in laboratory test tubes, or in animal models of MS, all become applied in the clinic to help us translate such fundamental disease information into studies of people with MS. Clinical trials (see Chapter 7) focus on testing the safety and efficacy of new drugs and agents developed to treat MS and its symptoms.

Another important area of clinical research is refinement and development of new techniques for diagnosis. Such techniques can be used to follow disease progress, particularly the relatively new "imaging" techniques that allow direct observation of lesions in the brain and spinal cord [magnetic resonance imaging (MRI) and related technologies]. New developments in analysis of blood, cerebrospinal fluid, and urine also have importance in diagnosis and in following the results of experimental clinical studies.

While new treatments are being developed to help reduce the symptoms and progression of MS, helping individuals and their families cope with the disease is an essential aspect of research in the areas of psychosocial studies, and health care delivery and policy research. Understanding the psychological and emotional aspects of MS has become a major focus of research in recent years, as we realize that brain pathology (as well as day-to-day stress) of the disease creates problems in cognitive (intellectual) and affective (emotional) function. Increased information in these areas is leading to new techniques to help with coping and rehabilitation, as well as specific interventions that can be applied in a clinical setting.

Although not limited to MS, the problems of access to care and services for people with chronic disease are increasingly becoming the focus of high quality health care delivery and policy research. Data gathered from such studies have a direct impact on altering public perception of chronic disease and on changing for the better legislative policy, entitlement programs, and societal policy for all people with disabilities.

Research in MS is broad-based and comprehensive, involving all aspects of basic and applied sciences related to biomedicine. Funding for this research has traditionally come from governmental agencies and multiple sclerosis societies in many countries around the world and more recently from pharmaceutical and biotechnology companies.

The results to date have been a significantly increased understanding of the disease, new and specific therapies, and significantly enhanced quality of life for people with MS. Basic and applied research are needed more than ever before to close the gaps in our knowledge of MS and move us closer to full treatment, prevention, and cure.

8

Searching for Treatments: The "Ins" and "Outs" of Clinical Trials

RESEARCH ON MANY FRONTS RELATED TO MS IS AN ACTIVE and vigorous undertaking. In the long run, all biomedical research in MS—be it the most basic or the most applied— is intended to gather information about the underlying disease process and is ultimately directed toward developing new therapeutics that may be safe and effective. Testing new drugs or devices developed through basic and clinical research is itself a major focus of MS research. Outcomes of such research can be treatments that can alter the disease course, prevent the disease from occurring, or improve function in people who already have MS—the totality of which would be a functional "cure" for MS. The ultimate research experiment, then, is the clinical trial.

A clinical trial is the scientific study of the efficacy and safety of a drug or device for a given disease on people who have that disease. As scientific studies, they are complex, time-consuming, and expensive, and must be done as carefully as any other scientific experiment to ensure that the study results are accurate, reproducible (repeatable by other scientists yielding the same results), and broadly applicable outside the original study population. Poorly done clinical trials that result in misleading conclusions are wasteful at best, and potentially dangerous for the intended population needing the treatment.

The Special Problems of MS Trials

PLACEBO EFFECT

While care must be taken to ensure the quality and integrity of any clinical trial, MS clinical trials are particularly difficult to undertake. One difficulty is the "placebo effect." People with MS are generally highly motivated to search for a treatment or cure for their disease, and this positive motivation can actually interfere with the objective assessment of any drug or device. This often occurs because of a phenomenon known as the placebo effect—the tendency to "improve" simply because of participation in a clinical trial, even if no active drug is being administered. A largely psychological phenomenon, the placebo effect is based in the faith that a given intervention will work, even if there is no evidence to support such faith. Working with a sympathetic physician who also strongly believes in the value of an experimental treatment can help to reinforce such tendencies.

Placebo effects likely have some true basis in the physiologic responses a person can have as a result of experiencing increased hope or excitement in the prospects of helping to find a truly useful therapy. These physiologic effects are poorly understood but can have an impact on sense of well-being and can even seem to cause improvement for a short time. This is particularly the case when measured results of treatment rely on self-reporting of symptoms or physical state by a treated patient rather than on the more rigorous objective assessment of performance by an examining physician or laboratory findings.

While important and potentially useful, such placebo effects must be carefully separated from a true therapeutic drug effect. In fact, any useful drug for MS must have an effect that is greater than the placebo effect.

MS NATURAL DISEASE VARIABILITY

The high degree of unpredictable variability in MS makes the design of clinical studies problematic. In any individual, the disease may go through seemingly spontaneous remissions and worsening, which are unpredictable in occurrence, severity, and duration. Spontaneous stabilization in previously progressive disease or a spontaneous remission of symptoms could easily be confused with a drug effect in a treatment program, even if the drug is having no impact whatsoever.

The disease may be very different from individual to individual. While symptoms of MS can be cataloged, no two individuals experience the same problems in the same ways. Because of this variability, clinical trials for new treatments must include provisions to overcome the natural disease variability over time and among individuals. A true drug effect must be separable from the natural variability in disease course.

UNDERSTANDING THE PREDICTED DRUG EFFECT

Drugs and other agents tested for MS generally have a mode of action that is more or less understood, and it is based on that mode of action in relation to what we know about the disease that the agents are tested for therapeutic benefit and safety. Different drugs may have different effects on various MS disease types. Agents that may be predicted to alter the frequency or severity of acute attacks of MS may have no benefit on longer term progression of disease. Thus, such a study must include only individuals with well-defined disease relapses and no progression, or the results at the end of years of exploration will be uninterpretable. By the same token, results of a study testing the ability of an agent to stop progression of disease would be muddied by the inclusion of patients with relapsing-remitting disease and no progression.

In the end, trials must be designed to answer questions on the particular type of disease or symptom for which the new agent is predicted to have an effect. Inclusion of individuals with different disease types or without the appropriate symptom problem may result in an incorrect conclusion.

Finally, some drugs may seem to cause improvement, but actually only have indirect effects on the disease. Agents with psychotropic effects, such as antidepressants, can help enormously in day-to-day coping with MS for patients who have depression associated with their disease, and such individuals will likely feel and perform better. This could be mistaken for an effect of the medication on the underlying disease process, when there really is none at all. Understanding the true effect of any drug on the disease process requires a detailed knowledge of the drug's action as well as careful clinical assessment of effects on the disease.

These and other problems associated with clinical trials can best be overcome by extremely rigorous experimental design for the studies. The generally accepted methods of study are time-consuming and expensive, but they hold the best chance of obtaining a clear-cut answer as to the efficacy and safety of any agent in MS.

MS Clinical Trial Study Design

SCIENTIFIC RATIONALE: A PRIMARY REQUIREMENT

The first step, and perhaps the most essential, in consideration of any new drug or agent for its therapeutic potential in MS is that it should have a strong scientific rationale for being tested in MS. Based on our knowledge of the MS process and on experimental studies of the drug in the laboratory, in animal disease models for MS, or in human disorders with similarities to MS, a physician/scientist will conclude that the drug may have a potential role in the treatment or management of MS. Drugs or any other substance or device without a scientific rationale related to the cause of MS should not even be considered for disease testing, since they will likely have no impact on disease outcome and will be wasteful of the time and effort of participating individuals with MS and their physicians, as well as the financial resources required for the study. Many "alternative therapies" can be faulted on this first criterion: a lack of bona fide rationale for even being considered in a disease such as MS.

PRELIMINARY OR "PHASE 1" STUDIES

Given a strong scientific rationale from basic and laboratory animal research, human trials almost always begin with toxicity or safety studies in a very small number of people with the disease (called a "preliminary" or "phase 1" clinical trial). In such early experiments, physicians usually have little sense of whether or not the candidate agent is safe for use in humans—the most vital consideration in any medical intervention. In these earliest studies, usually only a few very seriously ill people are asked to participate, since these people may find the potential risk of any new agent to be worthwhile, given the grave nature of their disease. If such studies demonstrate that the agent is safe, a physician may pursue further studies to get a sense of possible efficacy.

PILOT OR "PHASE 2" CLINICAL TRIALS

"Pilot" or "phase 2" studies usually involve larger, statistically relevant numbers of patients (often 20–100 or more) with a disease type and severity that seem appropriate to the known or hypothesized drug effect. Key issues in such a study are (1) determining the effectiveness of the drug in halting progression, reducing relapse rate, or improving symptoms and function; (2) obtaining additional information about toxicity and safety; and (3) refining knowledge about the best possible dose and route of delivery (i.e., oral, by injection, etc.).

Such pilot studies aim to be objective in obtaining the required answers. Thus, patient performance on drug may be compared to pre-drug status (so-called "longitudinal studies"), but, even better, should be compared to an identical group of patients who are on a "parallel track" but obtaining sham or placebo treatment—a treatment that looks identical to the actual drug or therapy but is therapeutically inactive. Because MS can change over time, even with no treatment intervention, "longitudinal studies" are usually unsatisfactory at this stage since it is impossible to know whether changes during the trial are due to the test drug or to underlying disease changes that may have occurred anyway.

True objectivity and elimination of placebo effects are enhanced if both the patients and the physicians who periodically check for efficacy are "blinded." In other words, neither knows which group of patients is on the real drug and which group is being given sham treatment. Double-blinded studies are hard to achieve, given the fact that many test agents have side effects that may be "unblinding" to the patient or examining physician, but rigorous efforts at blinding are essential to reduce the likelihood of false results due to placebo effects.

Results from such "phase 2" studies, which can often take several years to obtain, may or may not show statistical benefit to people on drug compared with people on sham therapy, as well as acceptable levels of side effects. If there is no benefit, or if there are uncontrollable or dangerous side effects, the agent is usually abandoned as a possible therapy. On the other hand, if benefit is indicated and side effects are minimal or acceptable, a further, larger clinical trial will be undertaken to confirm and expand the studies.

DEFINITIVE OR "PHASE 3" CLINICAL TRIALS

Definitive or "phase 3" trials are usually the final step toward making a decision about the value of a proposed therapy. As in the previous trial stage, the key questions concern efficacy and safety. Large, statistically determined numbers of participants are essential, and the study is often conducted at a number of different sites (so-called "multicenter") to ensure that the drug can be used in an equivalent fashion by many physicians. Rigorous adherence to blinding of patients and examining physicians, as well as careful random assignment of patients into treatment and sham groups, is essential to ensure objectivity. At the conclusion of the study period, when the blinding code is broken and the performance of drug-treated patients can be compared with the sham-treated group, there should be sufficient information to determine if the tested agent is truly safe and effective.

Recent definitive clinical trials for MS have included as many as 900 individuals, 40 participating centers, and have taken multiple years to complete. These are the "gold standard" studies from which physicians and patients may have the best confidence that the results are sound.

There are variations in the outlined studies, often depending on the amount of information available about a new drug from the laboratory, from use in other diseases, or from prior use in MS. Not all new agents go through a test phase in animal models of MS (Betaseron® did not because significant amounts of safety data from humans with other diseases were already in hand), and in some cases "phase 2" and "phase 3" studies are combined into a single large "phase 2/3" study when sufficient information is available from previous studies on dosing and route of delivery. However, the elements and data described are required to determine true benefit and safety. These are also the elements and data required by the U.S. Food and Drug Administration and similar regulatory bodies in many countries, which closely monitor clinical trials at every step. It is ultimately the regulatory authority's assessment of the efficacy and safety data and the care with which a study is done that determines whether any agent may be marketed as a treatment for MS.

POST-MARKETING OR "PHASE 4" STUDIES

Once governmental regulatory approval has been granted and the agent can be marketed and advertised as a treatment for MS, there is often a series of further studies, which are termed "postmarket" or "phase 4" studies. These are usually designed to collect information on further adverse reactions to the agent, to explore the use of the drug for different forms of disease (for instance, an approved drug for progressive MS might be tested in relapsing-remitting disease in a phase 4 analysis), or to test the effects of the drug on related disorders (for example, testing the efficacy and safety of a drug approved for MS on rheumatoid arthritis).

In some cases, regulatory authorities mandate phase 4 studies to collect data that were "missing" in the definitive analysis and which are important in understanding the use of the new medication. Sometimes the outcome of these mandated phase 4 studies can determine continued marketability of new agents. Should data become available that change the original understanding of the safety and efficacy of the new agent and compromise its use, regulatory authorities may have the obligation to remove the treatment from the market.

Financing Clinical Trials

Drug studies are time-consuming and expensive. Such studies are most often supported financially by pharmaceutical and biotechnological companies that invest significant "research and development" resources in these experiments. Grants from the federal government or voluntary health agencies, such as the National Multiple Sclerosis Society, also may fund part or all of the cost of clinical trials. It is rare (and often considered unethical) to request that a patient who volunteers to participate as an experimental subject be asked to pay for that privilege.

Who Participates in Clinical Trials?

The decision for any person with MS to participate in an experimental clinical trial is an intensely personal one and is highly subjective. Since there is always the potential for risk of any untested agent, a potential study participant must be fully informed by the treating physician, who must include a clear assessment of the potential risk factor in any information provided about the study. Informed consent, including close personal discussion with the physician and nurse as well as required written permission from the study participant, are legal requirements that protect the rights of all participants.

Not everyone really wants to participate in a clinical trial. Potential risk is one concern. Additionally, since good studies may require a sham treatment group, some people may balk at the possibility of volunteering to be in a study and then having a chance of being in the sham group, in which, for the duration of the study, he or she will receive inactive treatment without knowing it. A true sense of altruism, coupled with a sense of adventure, often characterizes those who volunteer to participate in such studies, since participation in either treatment or sham group may ultimately help tens of thousands of people with MS. The clinical trial volunteer is a real pioneer and a true hero.

Why Can't Some Patients Participate in Clinical Trials?

One of the most unfortunate dilemmas occurs when a person decides that he or she wants to participate in a clinical trial and finds that it is impossible. A frequently asked question is, "Doctor, why can't I be in your clinical trial?"

Clinical trials are limited in practice to a relatively small number of individuals who must be located geographically close to the clinical center(s) where the study is undertaken. Since most studies require intense clinic visits at specific predetermined times throughout several years, difficulties in travel from home to the clinic may be considered in whether or not someone will be accepted in a study.

The design of trials is such that generally only one type of MS—say, relapsing-remitting disease—is involved in the study. This excludes people with any other form of disease. Even within the group of interest, further restrictions—called inclusion and exclusion criteria—may be enforced in almost all studies: disease limited to a certain duration or a certain level of disability; restricted age of participants; exclusions based on prior medications or participation in previous trials where there might be dangerous or confusing effects with the new experimental treatment.

For any particular test drug, other restrictions may also apply, depending on the known characteristics of the test medication. There may be prohibitions against pregnancy if an agent is known to cause potential fetal harm; individuals with other medical conditions not related to MS that may be affected by known characteristics of the test medication may be excluded. These practical factors can often result in an eager patient's being refused a place in a new clinical trial.

If this should be the case, potential participants may take some solace from the realization that positive findings from a clinical trial will eventually benefit many, many more people than could ever hope to participate in the initial studies. Everyone will benefit from the time and effort invested by the few.

Where Can I Learn About Ongoing Clinical Trials?

Finding out about clinical trials in MS should be a joint project of the patient and the physician. The network of physicians who organize and run studies in MS is ever-growing, and in consultation with a personal physician, an interested patient can usually learn of any pending studies locally or nearby, often with the assistance of the local branch or chapter of the National Multiple Sclerosis Society or Multiple Sclerosis Society of Canada, or their over thirty affiliated member organizations around the world.

In summary, the ultimate research in MS is the development and testing of new therapies for use in the disease. Clinical trials designed to objectively test efficacy and safety are difficult and expensive to undertake. While people with MS are always needed to participate in such research, the decision to volunteer is often a difficult and personal one, and the practical restrictions involved in conducting clinical trials in MS often exclude many who would gladly participate. In the end, basic and clinical scientists, patients who participate in clinical trials, pharmaceutical companies and governmental and voluntary health agencies focused on MS worldwide are all partners in assuring the development of new treatments for individuals affected by MS.

9

How the National Multiple Sclerosis Society Can Help

PEOPLE WITH MULTIPLE SCLEROSIS (MS) HAVE NEEDS AND concerns relative to their diagnosis, many of which are shared by family members and close friends. The issues vary for each individual according to time since diagnosis, degree of impairment, and family and work situations. Other factors such as personality characteristics, previous life events, and learning and coping styles also have an impact. The family physician or neurologist is a frequent source of information. While this is certainly appropriate, a medical practice is not an adequate resource to accommodate the extensive non-medical needs of those with MS, their families, friends, and other concerned persons such as employers, teachers, and health professionals. The primary resource for addressing non-medical MS-related needs is the National Multiple Sclerosis Society. This chapter provides general information about the U.S. and Canadian Societies, as well as the specific ways the National MS Society (U.S.) can help you.

Overview of the National Multiple Sclerosis Society

The National Multiple Sclerosis Society (NMSS) is the only non-profit organization in the United States that supports national and international research on the prevention, cure, and treatment of MS, with more than $160 million expended to date. Equally important, the Society's goals include the provision of nationwide services to assist people with MS and their families and the provision of information about MS to those with the disease, family members, professionals, and the public. Programs are designed to help individuals maintain their independence and lifestyle, with "state of the art" health care and other support systems available. The Society's mission—to end the devastating effects of MS—addresses the negative impact of the disease in the present through education and services and into the future through research and advocacy.

The Society was founded in 1946 by Sylvia Lawry, whose brother had multiple sclerosis. In her search to learn more about the disease, she found that only two scientists in the country professed any interest in the disease. Ms. Lawry placed an advertisement in the *New York Times* seeking any information about successful treatments for MS. A number of people who were also touched by MS responded. They had no news of a cure, but asked that Ms. Lawry share whatever helpful information she received. And so the National MS Society was born. It has grown to more than 460,000 members, including over 218,000 people who have MS. People throughout the United States are reached by a system of 138 chapters and branches. These local units provide varying levels of assistance and education. The home office in New York City directs MS-related research and advocacy, provides some specific services, and provides support, structure, and guidance for chapters. Policies and national priorities are established by a National Board of Directors, composed of business and professional leaders with a special interest in MS. The Board is assisted by a nationally representative group of individuals with MS, the National Services Advisory Council. Each local chapter is governed by a Board of Trustees. Staff at both national and chapter levels work in partnership with volunteers and the community to implement the necessary and desired programs. There is an ongoing process of identifying needs and eliciting feedback regarding the value of programs. This involves people with MS, their families, and the professionals who serve them, and provides direction for Society activities.

Philosophy of Services

The NMSS and its chapters are committed to empowering people with MS to live as independently as possible within the limits of their disabilities, and to the maximum of their capabilities within the least restrictive environment. This goal is achieved through programs, services, and activities that:

- promote and support knowledge, health, and independence;
- provide information, education, and emotional support to help people with MS and their families help themselves;
- help people gain access to community resources;
- stimulate changes in the community and/or the development of new community resources/services beneficial to people affected by MS; and
- fill gaps in community resources.

The Society believes that all people with MS and their families in the United States should have access to basic services and is implementing this through its newly created "Nationwide Services Program."

All people with MS are offered services without discrimination, Access is not affected by a person's race, color, religion, age, disability, or sexual orientation, or the individual's relationship with a chapter. Chapters do hold "targeted" programs to meet the needs of specific groups, e.g., education programs for those newly diagnosed, young professionals' groups, gay/lesbian network, etc.

The confidentiality of members with MS ("clients") is strictly maintained. Client status is indistinguishable on the general membership list, and clients receive general Society mailings, including solicitations for support, unless a clear request to the contrary is made.

Who Are Served?

The Society's mission reflects our dedication to end the devastating effects of multiple sclerosis. The main recipients of chapter services are people who have multiple sclerosis. But others are also affected, so the secondary focus is the "family circle"—spouses, children, parents, relatives, significant others, coworkers, and close friends.

The NMSS is the leading source of information on multiple sclerosis for the general public. It also provides education to health professionals, service providers, and community agencies. Although not a direct service to people with MS or their families, such information and education can have significant impact on quality of life, increasing access to quality health care and community resources and promoting understanding from others.

Quality of Life Goals

The NMSS organizes services under three main Quality of Life Goals: MS Knowledge, Health, and Independence. Specific services are addressed within this framework.

Knowledge	*Health*	*Independence*
• Knowledge of MS by clients, families, professionals, the public	• Physical health • Emotional health • Family and social support	• Independent living • Accessibility • Employment • Long-term services

KNOWLEDGE

The National Multiple Sclerosis Society facilitates acquisition of essential knowledge about MS by providing information and education to clients, families, professionals, and the public.

Knowledge of MS by Clients and Families, Professionals, and the Public

Information about multiple sclerosis is the first and most frequent request the NMSS receives from people with MS. Client surveys consistently request more information about MS: symptoms, diagnosis, programs, treatment, research, and related issues such as employment, health insurance, disability rights, and family issues.

Seeking information about MS is usually a first step in the coping process. Getting accurate up-to-date information can assist you to make informed decisions, become aware of needs and resources, and take some control over an unpredictable and complex disease. One of the main functions of the NMSS is to serve as the repository of the most current and accurate information on MS.

- National information line (recording) through the Society's Information Resource Center (IRC) at 800-FIGHT-MS. Following selection of the IRC option, a recorded voice requests the topic of interest and mailing information.

- National information line (manned) through the IRC from 10:00 A.M. to 6:00 P.M., Monday through Friday, by calling 800-227-3166.
- Toll-free access to your local chapter by selecting the appropriate option at 800-FIGHT-MS.
- Internet Web site with updated information about treatments, current research, and programs (http://www,nmss.org); local home page in many areas.
- Knowledge Is Power educational program (serial mailings) for people *newly diagnosed* with MS and their families, available through most chapters.
- Moving Forward group educational program for people newly diagnosed with MS and their families, available through most chapters.
- Education programs on various topics throughout the year.
- Annual national teleconference at over 500 sites throughout the United States on three Saturdays in May; call your chapter for the location nearest you.
- Booklets, articles, and information sheets on MS-related topics (see "Resource Guide").
- Lending library of books, audio- and/or videotapes, with mail access, through your local chapter.
- *Inside MS* national quarterly magazine, and chapter newsletter quarterly or more often.

HEALTH

The National Multiple Sclerosis Society helps people with MS to achieve optimal health physically, emotionally, and in their relationships.

Physical Health

People with multiple sclerosis must deal with concerns about physical impairments related to the disease and their impact on general physical health. NMSS programs and services address physical health needs by:

- Promoting "state of the art" *MS healthcare* and facilitating access for people with MS;

- Providing *referrals to neurologists,* physical therapists, and other medical/rehabilitation professionals knowledgeable about MS;
- *Swimming and other exercise programs* sponsored or co-sponsored by some chapters, or referral to existing programs in the community
- *Wellness programs* in some chapters.
- Affiliation with local *MS clinical facilities* to facilitate access to, and coordination of, physical health services.
- Participation in *local and national advocacy* issues related to physical health, e.g.,health insurance reform, through *Action Alert Network.* (call your local chapter to join).

Emotional Health

Emotional health is a state of psychological well-being, which includes the individual's adaptive capacities. It is demonstrated by successful interactions with others and with the social environment. Difficulties with adaptation in a chronic illness are normal and respond favorably to a variety of interventions.

Although NMSS chapters are not primarily mental health agencies, we can help individuals and their significant others in their adaptation to chronic illness. Chapters provide short-term counseling, defined as "reflective listening and problem solving." The social isolation that often results from having a chronic illness can be reduced through peer relationships and group programs that bring people together.

Assistance with problem solving:

- local counselor/therapist referrals
- self-help groups—leaders have often received group leadership training through the Society
- COPE newsletter to self-help groups

Family and Social Support

Families of people with MS are important to the National MS Society, which has formally adopted the Family Service America, Inc. definition of family: "A family consists of two or more people, whether living together or apart, related by blood, marriage, adoption, or commitment to care for one another."

This definition highlights the inclusion of all varieties of family configurations. The NMSS recognizes the enormous, ongoing stress that the entire family experiences, as well as the critical support provided by the family to the member with MS. Programs emphasize the strengths of the family and bolster these strengths by offering education and other means of support and assistance.

- "Someone to Listen" peer counseling program, which meets the second most requested service—to speak with another person who has MS. "Peers" are specially trained to provide information and support to the person with MS;
- family one-day programs combining education, counseling, and social activities (in some chapters);
- social events such as holiday parties;
- "Children with MS" program, which matches children/teens with MS appropriate peers and offers parents the opportunity to network (call the NY Home Office: 212-476-0457).
- family counseling programs in some chapters, referrals to experienced community counselors in others.

INDEPENDENCE

The National Multiple Sclerosis Society is committed to promoting the highest possible level of independence for people with MS. This category of programs and services does not deal with the immediate needs of people recently diagnosed, but does look at some of the long-term issues of which we all should be aware.

Independent Living

Referrals to centers for independent living, equipment vendors, accessible housing, and others.

Accessibility

All chapter offices and program locations are accessible to people with disabilities.

Employment

Referrals and consultations to help people continue employment despite MS-related obstacles.

Long-Term Services

Programs to help people who are moderately to severely limited by MS-related disability receive necessary personal services and other assistance.

The Multiple Sclerosis Society of Canada

Founded in 1948, the Multiple Sclerosis Society of Canada has a membership of 27,000, with seven regional divisions and more than 130 chapters. The Head Office is located in Toronto, Ontario. Division offices are located in Dartmouth, Montreal, Toronto, Winnipeg, Regina, Edmonton, and Vancouver. The mission is "to be a leader in finding a cure for multiple sclerosis and enabling people affected by MS to enhance their quality of life." The Multiple Sclerosis Society of Canada expends more than $4 million annually on medical research programs.

INDIVIDUAL AND FAMILY SERVICES

The Multiple Sclerosis Society of Canada provides a wide variety of services for people who have MS and their families:

- supportive counseling;
- referral;
- self-help groups;
- ASK MS Information System;
- educational workshops;
- equipment program;
- social and recreational activities;
- information about MS for health care professionals;
- network of specialized MS clinics.

Services vary across the country depending on the kind of provincial government and community programs available, since the MS Society does not wish to duplicate services already in existence. The Society currently spends more than $4 million annually on services and education programs for people who have MS, their family members, and health care professionals.

PUBLIC EDUCATION

The MS Society is firmly committed to informing Canadians about multiple sclerosis and how they can join the fight against MS. The national office coordinates an overall public awareness campaign that is supplemental and complemented by activities at the divisional and chapter levels.

SOCIAL ACTION

The Multiple Sclerosis Society of Canada has long been aware of its responsibility to bring about changes to government policies and private actions and attitudes that will positively benefit people with MS. Since December 1987, when the National Board of Directors approved the formation of the National Social Action Committee, Society volunteers have been pursuing these goals in a more coordinated manner.

FUND RAISING

The Multiple Sclerosis Society of Canada has total revenues of more than $17 million annually. The funds are used to support research, individual and family services, public education, social action, and volunteer resources. Most of this income comes from public donations, bequests, and special fund raising programs conducted by the MS Society. The five major fund raising programs are the MS Carnation Campaign, the MS Bike Tour, the MS Read-A-Thon, the Super Cities Walk for Multiple Sclerosis, and the Direct Mail Campaign.

HISTORY

The first multiple sclerosis society in the world—the National Multiple Sclerosis Society (USA)—began in 1946. After contact with the American organization, a small group of dedicated volunteers in Montreal founded the Multiple Sclerosis Society of Canada in 1948. Support of MS research began in 1949.

Headquarters for the Society remained in Montreal until the mid-1960s, when the offices were moved to Toronto. Other advances came with the establishment of regional divisions; there are now seven divisions across Canada, from coast to coast. The International Federation of Multiple Sclerosis Societies, of which the Canadian Society is a charter member, was established in 1967.

INDIVIDUAL AND FAMILY SERVICES SUMMARY CHART

Alberta Division	*Atlantic Division*	*British Columbia Division*
11203-70th Street	71 Ilsley Avenue	1130 West Pender Street
2nd Floor	Unit 12	16th Floor
Edmonton, AB	Dartmouth, NS	Vancouver, BC
T5B 1T1	B3B 1L5	V6E 4A4
403-471-3313	902-468-8230	604-689-3144

Manitoba Division
825 Sherbrook Street
2nd Floor
Winnipeg, MB
R3A 1M5
204-783-8585

Ontario Division
250 Bloor Street East
Suite 1000
Toronto, ON
M4W 3P9
416-922-6065

Quebec Division
666 Sherbrooke Street
  West, Suite 1500
Montreal, PQ
H3A 1E7
514-849-7592

Saskatchewan Division
2329-11th Avenue
Regina, SK
S4P 0K2
306-522-5607

Call toll-free in Canada 800-268-7582.

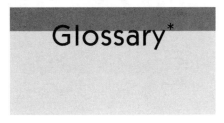

Glossary*

Activities of daily living (ADLs)

Activities of daily living include any daily activity a person performs for self-care (feeding, grooming, bathing, dressing), work, home-making, and leisure. The ability to perform ADLs is often used as a measure of ability/disability in MS.

Acute

Having rapid onset, usually with recovery; not chronic or long-lasting.

Antibodies

Proteins of the immune system that are soluble (dissolved) in blood serum or other body fluids and which are produced in response to bacteria,viruses, and other types of foreign antigens. *See* Antigen.

Anticholinergic

Refers to the action of certain medications commonly used in the management of neurogenic bladder dysfunction. These medications inhibit the transmission of parasympathetic nerve impulses and thereby reduce spasms of smooth muscle in the bladder.

Antigen

Any substance that triggers the immune system to produce an anti-body; generally refers to infectious or toxic substances. *See* Antibodies.

---

* This glossary addresses the specific needs of newly diagnosed people with MS. It is a brief version of the comprehensive glossary in *Multiple Sclerosis: The Questions You Have—The Answers You Need.* See "Additional Readings" for additional information.

Assistive devices

Any tools that are designed, fabricated, and/or adapted to assist a person in performing a particular task, e.g., cane, walker, shower chair, adapted kitchen utensils, etc.

Ataxia

The incoordination and unsteadiness that result from the brain's failure to regulate the body's posture and the strength and direction of limb movements. Ataxia is most often caused by disease activity in the cerebellum.

Autoimmune disease

An immune system malfunction in which the body's immune system causes illness by mistakenly attacking healthy cells, organs, or tissues in the body. Multiple sclerosis is believed to be an autoimmune disease, along with systemic lupus erythematosus, rheumatoid arthritis, scleroderma, and many others.

Autonomic nervous system

The part of the nervous system that regulates "involuntary" vital functions, including the activity of the cardiac (heart) muscle, smooth muscles (e.g., of the gut), and glands.

B-cell

A type of lymphocyte (white blood cell) manufactured in the bone marrow that makes antibodies.

Babinski reflex

A neurologic sign in MS in which stroking the outside sole of the foot with a pointed object causes an upward (extensor) movement of the big toe rather than the normal (flexor) bunching and downward movement of the toes. *See* Sign.

Blood-brain barrier

A semi-permeable cell layer around blood vessels in the brain and spinal cord that prevents large molecules, immune cells, and potentially damaging substances and disease-causing organisms (e.g., viruses) from passing out of the blood stream into the central nervous system (brain and spinal cord). A break in the blood-brain barrier may underlie the disease process in MS.

Brainstem

The part of the central nervous system that houses the nerve centers of the head as well as the centers for respiration and heart control. It extends from the base of the brain to the spinal cord.

Catheter, urinary

A hollow, flexible tube, made of plastic or rubber, which can be inserted through the urinary opening into the bladder to drain excess urine that cannot be excreted normally.

Central nervous system

The part of the nervous system that includes the brain, optic nerves, and spinal cord.

Cerebellum

A part of the brain situated above the brainstem that controls balance and coordination of movement.

Cerebrospinal fluid (CSF)

A watery, colorless, clear fluid that bathes and protects the brain and spinal cord. The composition of this fluid can be altered by a variety of diseases. Certain changes in CSF that are characteristic of MS can be detected with a lumbar puncture (spinal tap), a test sometimes used to help make the MS diagnosis.

Cerebrum

The large, upper part of the brain, which acts as a master control system and is responsible for initiating thought and motor activity.

Clinical finding

An observation made during a medical examination indicating change or impairment in a physical or mental function.

Clonus

A sign of spasticity in which involuntary shaking or jerking of the leg occurs when the toe is placed on the floor with the knee slightly bent. The shaking is caused by repeated, rhythmic, reflex muscle contractions.

Cognition

High level functions carried out by the human brain, including comprehension and formation of speech, visual perception and construction, calculation ability, attention (information processing), memory, and executive functions such as planning, problem-solving, and self-monitoring.

Cognitive impairment

Changes in cognitive function caused by trauma or disease process. Some degree of cognitive impairment occurs in approximately 50–60 percent of people with MS, with memory, information processing, and executive functions being the most commonly affected functions.

Cognitive rehabilitation

Techniques designed to improve the functioning of individuals whose cognition is impaired because of physical trauma or disease. Rehabilitation strategies are designed to improve the impaired function via repetitive drills or practice, or to compensate impaired functions that are not likely to improve. Cognitive rehabilitation is provided by psychologists and neuropsychologists, speech/language pathologists, and occupational therapists. While these three types of specialists use different assessment tools and treatment strategies, they share the common goal of improving the individual's ability to function as independently and safely as possible in the home and work environment.

Computerized axial tomography (CAT scan)

A non-invasive diagnostic radiology technique. A computer integrates X-ray scanned "slices" of the organ being examined into a cross-sectional picture.

Contraction

A shortening of muscle fibers and muscle that produce movement around a joint.

Coordination

An organized working together of muscles and groups of muscles aimed at bringing about a purposeful movement such as walking or standing.

Corticosteroids

See ACTH, Glucocorticoid hormones.

Cortisone

A glucocorticoid steroid hormone, produced by the adrenal glands or synthetically, that has anti-inflammatory and immune-system suppressing properties. Prednisone and prednisolone also belong to this group of substances used in MS to decrease the duration of attacks.

Cranial nerves

Nerves that carry sensory or motor fibers to the face and neck. Included among this group of twelve nerves are the optic nerve (vision), trigeminal nerve (sensation along the face), vagus nerve (pharynx and vocal cords). Evaluation of cranial nerve function is part of the standard neurologic exam.

Deep tendon reflexes

The involuntary jerks that are normally produced at certain spots on a limb when the tendons are tapped with a hammer. Reflexes are tested as part of the standard neurological exam.

Demyelination

A loss of myelin in the white matter of the nervous system.

Diplopia

Double vision, or the simultaneous awareness of two images of the same object that results from a failure of the two eyes to work in a coordinated fashion. Covering one eye will erase one of the images.

Disability

As defined by the World Health Organization, a disability (resulting from an impairment) is a restriction or lack of ability to perform an activity in the manner or within the range considered normal for a human being.

Double-blind clinical study

A study in which none of the participants, including experimental subjects, examining doctors, attending nurses, or any other research staff, know who is taking the test drug and who is taking a control or placebo agent. The purpose of this research design is to avoid inadvertent bias of the test results. In all studies, procedures are designed to "break the blind" if medical circumstances require it.

Dysesthesia

Distorted or unpleasant sensations experienced by a person when the skin is touched.

Electroencephalography (EEG)

A diagnostic procedure that records, via electrodes attached to various areas of the person's head, electrical activity generated by brain cells.

Electromyography (EMG)

A diagnostic procedure that records muscle electrical potentials through electrodes.

Etiology

The study of all factors that may be involved in the development of a disease, including the patient's susceptibility, the nature of the disease-causing agent, and the way in which the person's body is invaded by the agent.

Evoked potentials (EPs)

Recordings of the nervous system's electrical response to the stimulation of specific sensory pathways (e.g., visual, auditory, general sensory). EPs can demonstrate lesions along specific nerve pathways whether or not the lesions are producing symptoms, thus making this test useful in confirming the diagnosis of MS.

Exacerbation

The appearance of new symptoms or the aggravation of old ones (synonymous with attack, relapse, flare-up, or worsening); usually associated with inflammation and demyelination in the brain or spinal cord.

Experimental allergic encephalomyelitis (EAE)

An autoimmune disease resembling MS that is induced in genetically susceptible research animals. Before testing on humans, a potential treatment for MS may first be tested on laboratory animals with EAE in order to determine the treatment's efficacy and safety.

Extensor spasm

A symptom of spasticity in which the legs straighten suddenly into a stiff, extended position. These spasms, which typically last for several minutes, occur most commonly in bed at night or on rising from bed.

Flaccid

A decrease in muscle tone resulting in weakened muscles and therefore loose, "floppy" limbs.

Flexor spasm

Involuntary, sometimes painful contractions of the flexor muscles, which pull the legs upward into a clenched position. They often occur during sleep, but can also occur when the person is in a seated position.

Food and Drug Administration (FDA)

The U.S. federal agency that is responsible for establishing and enforcing governmental regulations pertaining to the manufacture and sale of food, drugs, and cosmetics. Its role is to certify benefits of medication and prevent the sale of impure or dangerous substances. Any new drug that is proposed for the treatment of MS must be approved by the FDA.

Foot drop

A condition of weakness in the muscles of the foot and ankle, caused by poor nerve conduction, which interferes with a person's ability to flex the ankle and walk with a normal heel-toe pattern. The toes touch the ground before the heel, causing the person to trip or lose balance.

Frontal lobes

The anterior (front) part of each of the cerebral hemispheres that make up the cerebrum. The back part of the frontal lobe is the motor cortex, which controls voluntary movement; the area of the frontal lobe that is further forward is concerned with learning, behavior, judgment, and personality.

Glucocorticoid hormones

Steroid hormones that are produced by the adrenal glands in response to stimulation by adrenocorticotropic hormone (ACTH) from the pituitary. These hormones, which can also be manufactured synthetically (prednisone, prednisolone, methylprednisolone, betamethasone, dexamethasone), serve both an immunosuppressive and an anti-inflammatory role in the treatment of MS exacerbations: they help control overactive immune response and interfere with the release of certain inflammation-producing enzymes.

Handicap

As defined by the World Health Organization, a handicap is a disadvantage, resulting from an impairment and disability, that interferes with a person's efforts to fulfill a role that is normal for that person. Handicap is therefore a social concept, representing the social and environmental consequences of a person's impairments and disabilities.

Helper T-lymphocytes

White blood cells that are a major contributor to the immune system's inflammatory response against myelin.

Immune system

A complex system of cells and dissolvable proteins that protect the body against disease-producing organisms and other foreign invaders.

Immunocompetent cells

White blood cells (B- and T-lymphocytes and others) that defend against invading agents in the body.

Immunosuppression

In MS, a form of treatment that slows or inhibits the body's natural immune responses, including those directed against the body's own tissues. Examples of immunosuppressive treatments in MS include cycloposphamide, cyclosporine, methotrexate, and azathioprine.

Impairment

As defined by the World Health Organization, an impairment is any loss of function directly resulting from injury or disease.

Incidence

The number of new cases of a disease in a specified population over a defined period of time.

Incontinence

The inability to control passage of urine or feces.

Inflammation

A tissue's immunologic response to injury, characterized by mobilization of white blood cells and antibodies, swelling, and fluid accumulation.

Intention tremor

Rhythmic shaking that occurs in the course of a purposeful movement, such as reaching to pick something up or bringing an outstretched finger in to touch one's nose.

Interferon

A group of immune system proteins, produced and released by cells infected by a virus, which inhibit viral multiplication by modifying the body's immune response. Several interferons have approved by the Food and Drug Administration for treatment of relapsing-remitting MS.

Lumbar puncture

A diagnostic procedure that uses a hollow needle to penetrate the spinal canal to remove cerebrospinal fluid for analysis. This procedure is used to examine the cerebrospinal fluid for changes in composition that are characteristic of MS (e.g., elevated white cell count, elevated protein content).

Lymphocyte

A type of white blood cell that is part of the immune system. Lymphocytes can be subdivided into two main groups: B-lymphocytes, which originate in the bone marrow and produce antibodies; T-lymphocytes, which are produced in the bone marrow and mature in the thymus. Helper T-lymphocytes heighten immune responses; suppressor T-lymphocytes suppress them and seem to be in short supply during an MS exacerbation.

Macrophage

A white blood cell with scavenger characteristics that ingests and destroys foreign substances, such as bacteria and cell debris.

Magnetic resonance imaging (MRI)

A diagnostic procedure that produces visual images of body parts without the use of X-rays. An important diagnostic tool in MS, MRI makes it possible to visualize and count lesions in the white matter of the brain and spinal cord.

Minimal Record of Disability (MRD)

A standardized method for quantifying the clinical status of a person with MS. The MRD is made up of five parts: demographic information; the Neurological Functional Systems, which assign scores to clinical findings for each of the various neurologic systems in the brain and spinal cord (pyramidal, cerebellar, brainstem, sensory, visual, mental, bowel and bladder); the Disability Status Scale, which gives a single composite score for the person's disease; the Incapacity Status Scale, which is an inventory of functional disabilities relating to activities of daily living; the Environmental Status Scale, which provides an assessment of social handicap resulting from chronic illness. The MRD assist doctors and other professionals in assessing the impact of MS and in planning and coordinating the care of people with MS.

Monoclonal antibodies

Laboratory-produced antibodies, which can be designed to react against a specific antigen in order to alter the immune response.

Motor neurons

Nerve cells of the brain and spinal cord that enable movement of muscles in various parts of the body.

Muscle tone

A characteristic of a muscle brought about by the constant flow of nerve stimuli to that muscle. Abnormal muscle tone can be defined as: hypertonus (increased muscle tone, as in spasticity); hypotonus (reduced muscle tone (flaccid paralysis); atony (loss of muscle tone). Muscle tone is evaluated as part of the standard neurologic exam in MS.

Myelin

A fatty white coating of nerve fibers in the central nervous system, composed of lipids (fats) and protein. Myelin serves as insulation and as an aid to efficient nerve fiber conduction. When myelin is damaged in MS, nerve fiber conduction is faulty or absent.

Myelin basic protein

A protein comprising about 30 percent of all myelin of the central nervous system that may be found in higher than normal concentrations in the cerebrospinal fluid of individuals with MS and other diseases that damage myelin. Some believe myelin basic protein is an antigen against which autoimmune responses are triggered in MS.

Myelitis

An inflammatory disease of the spinal cord. In transverse myelitis, the inflammation spreads across the tissue of the spinal cord, resulting in a loss of its normal function to transmit nerve impulses up and down, as though the spinal cord had been severed.

Nerve

A bundle of nerve fibers (axons). Fibers are either afferent (leading toward the brain and serving in the perception of sensory stimuli of the skin, joints, muscles, and inner organs) or efferent (leading away from the brain and mediating contractions of muscles or organs).

Nervous system

Includes all of the neural structures in the body: the central nervous system consists of the brain, spinal cord, and optic nerves; the peripheral nervous system consists of the nerve roots and nerves throughout the body.

Neurogenic bladder

Bladder dysfunction associated with neurologic malfunction in the spinal cord and characterized by a failure to empty, failure to store, or a combination of the two. Symptoms that result from these three types of dysfunction include urinary urgency, frequency, hesitancy, nocturia, and incontinence.

Neurologist

Physician who specializes in the diagnosis and treatment of conditions related to the nervous system.

Neuron

The basic nerve cell of the nervous system. A neuron consists of a nucleus within a cell body and one or more processes (extensions) called dendrites and axons.

Occupational therapist (OT)

Occupational therapists assess functioning in activities of everyday living that are essential for independent living, including dressing, bathing, grooming, meal preparation, writing, and driving.

Oligoclonal bands

A diagnostic sign indicating abnormal levels of certain antibodies in the cerebrospinal fluid; seen in approximately 90 percent of people with multiple sclerosis, but not specific to MS.

Oligodendrocyte

A cell in the central nervous system that is responsible for making and supporting myelin.

Optic neuritis

Inflammation or demyelination of the optic (visual) nerve with transient or permanent impairment of vision and occasionally pain.

Orthosis

A mechanical appliance (such as a leg brace or splint) that is specially designed to control, correct, or compensate for impaired limb function.

Paresthesia

A sensation of burning, prickling, tingling, or creeping on the skin that is often seen in MS.

Paroxysmal symptoms

Symptoms that have sudden onset, apparently in response to some kind of movement or sensory stimulation, last for a few moments, and then subside. Paroxysmal symptoms tend to occur frequently in those individuals who have them, and follow a similar pattern from one episode to the next. Examples of paroxysmal symptoms include acute episodes of trigeminal neuralgia (sharp facial pain), tonic seizures (intense spasm of limb or limbs on one side of the body), dysarthria (slurred speech often accompanied by loss of balance and coordination), and various paresthesias (sensory disturbances ranging from tingling to severe pain).

Physiatrist

Physicians who specialize in the rehabilitation of physical impairments.

Physical therapist (PT)

Physical therapists evaluate and improve movement and function of the body, with particular attention to physical mobility, balance, posture, fatigue, and pain.

Placebo

An inactive compound designed to look just like a test drug in a clinical drug study as a means of assessing the benefits and liabilities of the test drug taken by experimental group subjects.

Placebo effect

An apparently beneficial result of therapy that occurs because of the patient's expectation that the therapy will help, in the absence of any real treatment.

Plaque

An area of inflamed or demyelinated central nervous system tissue.

Postural tremor

Rhythmic shaking that occurs when the muscles are tensed to hold an object or stay in a given position.

Prevalence

The number of all new and old cases of a disease in a defined population at a particular point in time.

Primary progressive MS

A clinical course of MS characterized from the beginning by progressive disease, with no plateaus or remissions, or an occasional plateau and very short-lived, minor improvements.

Prognosis

Prediction of the future course of the disease.

Pseudo-exacerbation

A temporary aggravation of disease symptoms, sometimes resulting from an elevation in body temperature or other stressor (e.g., an infection, severe fatigue, constipation), that disappears once the stressor is removed. A pseudo-exacerbation involves flare-ups of prior or existing symptoms rather than new disease activity or progression.

Pyramidal tracts

Motor nerve pathways in the brain and spinal cord that connect nerve cells in the brain to the motor cells located in the cranial, thoracic, and lumbar parts of the spinal cord. Damage to these tracts causes spastic paralysis or weakness.

Reflex

An involuntary response of the nervous system to a stimulus, such as the stretch reflex, which is elicited by tapping a tendon with a reflex hammer, resulting in a contraction. Increased, diminished, or absent reflexes can be indicative of neurologic damage, including MS, and are therefore tested as part of the standard neurologic exam.

Relapsing-remitting MS

A clinical course of MS that is characterized by clearly defined, acute attacks with full or partial recovery and no disease progression between attacks.

Remission

A lessening in the severity of symptoms or their temporary disappearance during the course of the illness.

Remyelination

The repair of damaged myelin. Myelin repair occurs spontaneously in MS but very slowly.

Sclerosis

Hardening of tissue. In MS, sclerosis is the replacement of lost myelin around CNS nerve cells with scar tissue.

Secondary progressive MS

A clinical course of MS that initially is relapsing-remitting and then becomes progressive at a variable rate, with or without relapses and remissions over a progressive course.

Sensory

Related to bodily sensations such as pain, smell, taste, temperature, vision, hearing, and position in space.

Sign

An objective physical problem or abnormality identified by the physician during the neurologic examination, including altered eye movements and other changes in the appearance or function of the visual system; altered reflexes; weakness; spasticity; sensory changes.

Spasticity

Abnormal increase in muscle tone, manifested as a spring-like resistance to moving or being moved.

Sphincter

A circular band of muscle fibers that tightens or closes a natural opening of the body, such as the external anal sphincter, which closes the anus, and the internal and external urinary sphincters, which close the urinary canal.

Steroids

See Glucocorticoid hormones.

Symptom

A subjectively perceived problem or complaint reported by the patient. In multiple sclerosis, common symptoms include visual problems, fatigue, sensory changes, weakness or paralysis of limbs, tremor, lack of coordination, poor balance, bladder or bowel changes, and psychological changes. *See* Sign.

Tonic seizure

An intense spasm that lasts for a few minutes and affects one or both limbs on one side of the body. Like other types of paroxysmal symptoms in MS, these spasms occur abruptly and fairly frequently in those individuals who have them, and are similar from one brief episode to the next. The attacks may be triggered by movement or occur spontaneously. *See* Paroxysmal symptom.

Trigeminal neuralgia

Lightning-like, acute pain in the face caused by demyelination of nerve fibers at the site where the sensory (trigeminal) nerve root for that part of the face enters the brainstem.

Urinary frequency

Perception of need or urge to urinate more frequently than normal due to small contracted bladder.

Urinary hesitancy

The inability to void urine spontaneously even though the urge to do so is present.

Urinary urgency

The inability to postpone urination once the need to void has been felt.

Vertigo

A dizzying sensation of the environment spinning, often accompanied by nausea and vomiting.

Additional Readings*

NOTE: *The Information Resource Center and Library of the National Multiple Sclerosis Society (800-344-4867) has a complete collection of booklets and articles about all aspects of MS research, treatments, and management. Operators are available to answer your questions and send you information on any MS-related topics that are of interest to you.*

Burnfield A (1985). *Multiple Sclerosis: A Personal Exploration.* New York: Demos.

Garee B (ed.) (1989). *Parenting: Tips from Parents (Who Happen to Have a Disability) on Raising Children.* Bloomington, IL: Accent Press.

Giffels JJ (1996). *Clinical Trials: What You Should Know Before Volunteering to Be a Research Subject.* New York: Demos Vermande.

James JL (1993). *One Particular Harbor: The Outrageous True Adventures of One Woman with Multiple Sclerosis Living in the Alaskan Wilderness.* Chicago: Noble Press.

Kalb RC (1996). *Multiple Sclerosis: The Questions You Have—The Answers You Need.* New York: Demos Vermande

Kalb RC, Scheinberg LC (1992). *Multiple Sclerosis and the Family.* New York: Demos.

Kraft GH, Catanzaro M (1996). *Living with Multiple Sclerosis: A Wellness Approach.* New York: Demos Vermande.

---

* This reading list addresses the specific needs of newly diagnosed people with MS. It is a brief version of the comprehensive resource list in *Multiple Sclerosis: The Questions You Have—The Answers You Need;* see above for details.

Lechtenberg R (1995). *Multiple Sclerosis Fact Book.* Philadelphia: Davis.

LeMaistre J (1994). *Beyond Rage: Mastering Unavoidable Health Changes.* Dillon, CO: Alpine Guild.

MacFarlane EB, Burstein P (1994). *Legwork: An Inspiring Journey Through a Chronic Illness.* New York: Charles Scribner's Sons.

Pitzele SK (1986). *We Are Not Alone: Learning to Live with Chronic Illness.* New York: Workman.

Register C (1987). *Living with Chronic Illness: Days of Patience and Passion.* New York: Free Press.

Rogers J, Matsumura M (1990). *Mother to Be: A Guide to Pregnancy and Birth for Women with Disabilities.* New York: Demos.

Rosner LJ, Ross S (1987). *Multiple Sclerosis: New Hope and Practical Guidelines for People with MS and Their Families.* New York: Prentice Hall.

Schapiro RT (1994). *Symptom Management in Multiple Sclerosis* (2nd edition). New York: Demos.

Scheinberg LC, Holland N (eds.) (1987). *Multiple Sclerosis: A Guide for Patients and Their Families.* New York: Raven.

Shuman R, Schwartz J (1988). *Understanding Multiple Sclerosis.* Riverside, NJ: Macmillan.

Sibley WA (1996). *Therapeutic Claims in Multiple Sclerosis* (4th edition). New York: Demos Vermande.

Webster B (1989). *All of a Piece: A Life with Multiple Sclerosis.* Baltimore: Johns Hopkins.

Wolf J (1987). *Mastering Multiple Sclerosis: A Guide to Management.* Rutland, VT: Academy Books.

Wolf J, Miles, M, Pickett K (1993). *Vignettes: Stories from Lives with Multiple Sclerosis.* Rutland, VT: Academy Books.

Wolf J (1991). *Fall Down Seven Times, Get Up Eight.* Rutland, VT: Academy Books.

Wright LM, Leahey M (1987). *Families and Chronic Illness.* Philadelphia: Spring House.

Zola IK (1982). *Missing Pieces: A Chronicle of Living with a Disability.* Philadelphia: Temple University Press.

NATIONAL MULTIPLE SCLEROSIS SOCIETY PUBLICATIONS
(212-986-3240; 800-344-4867)

Booklets:

- *Living with MS*—Debra Frankel, M.S., O.T.R., with Hettie Jones
- *What Everyone Should Know About Multiple Sclerosis*
- *Things I Wish Someone Had Told Me: Practical Thoughts for People Newly Diagnosed with Multiple Sclerosis*—Suzanne Rogers
- *Research Directions in Multiple Sclerosis*—Stephen C. Reingold, Ph.D.
- *ADA and People with MS*—Laura Cooper, Esq., Nancy Law, L.S.W., with Jane Sarnoff
- *Enhancing Productivity On Your Job: The Win-Win Approach*—Richard T. Roessler, Ph.D., and Phillip Rumrill, Ph.D.
- *The Rehab Outlook*—Lisa J. Bain and Randall T. Schapiro, M.D.
- *Food for Thought: MS and Nutrition*—Jane Sarnoff, with Daniel Kosich, Ph.D.
- *Multiple Sclerosis and Your Emotions*—Mary Eve Sanford, Ph.D., and Jack H. Petajan, M.D.
- *Solving Cognitive Problems*—Nicholas G. LaRocca, Ph.D., with Martha King
- *Understanding Bladder Problems in MS*—Nancy J. Holland, Ed.D., and Michele G. Madonna, R.N., M.A.
- *Understanding Bowel Problems in MS*—Nancy J. Holland, Ed.D., with Robin Frames.
- *Sexual Dysfunction*—Robin Frames
- *Moving with Multiple Sclerosis*—Iris Kimberg, M.S., O.T.R., R.P.T.
- *PLAINTALK: A Booklet About MS for Families*—Debra Frankel, M.S., O.T.R., and Sarah Minden, M.D.
- *Coping with Stress*—(adapted from material by the Arthritis Foundation), Philip Smith and staff at the Chicago-Greater Illinois Chapter
- *Someone You Know Has MS: A Book for Families*—Cyrisse Jaffee, Debra Frankel, Barbara LaRoche, and Patricia Dick
- *When a Parent Has MS: A Teenager's Guide*—Pamela Cavallo, M.S.W., with Martha Jablow

- *Taking Care: A Guide for Well Partners*—Nancy J. Holland, Ed.D., R.N., with Jane Sarnoff
- *Coping with Fatigue in MS Takes Understanding and Planning*—Alexander Burnfield, M.B., M.R.C. Psych.

Other MS Society Publications:

- *Facts and Issues* (reprints of articles that originally appeared in the National MS Society magazine, Inside MS, covering such topics as diagnosis, pregnancy, pain, gait problems, genes and MS susceptibility, fatigue, etc.)
- *Inside MS*—a 24-page magazine published three times yearly
- *Inside MS Bulletin*—an 8-page newsletter extracted from *Inside MS* (published three times a year)

Monograph Series (1995)

- *Families Affected by Multiple Sclerosis: Disease Impacts and Coping Strategies*—Rosalind C. Kalb, Ph.D.
- *Long-Term Care and Multiple Sclerosis*—Debra Frankel, M.S., O.T.R.
- *Employment and Multiple Sclerosis*—Nicholas G. LaRocca, Ph.D.
- *Economic Costs of Multiple Sclerosis: How Much and Who Pays*—Carol Harvey, Ph.D.
- *Utilization and Perceptions of Healthcare Services by People with MS*—Leon Sternfeld, M.D., Ph.D., M.P.H.

EASTERN PARALYZED VETERANS ASSOCIATION PUBLICATIONS
(800-444-0120)

- *Understanding the Americans with Disabilities Act* (English and Spanish)
- *The ADA: Resource Information Guide* (bibliography of books and videotapes)
- *Air Carrier Access* (defines the Air Carrier Access Act and gives information about air travel for wheelchair users)
- *Accessible Building Design* (a description of the essential components of an accessible building, including dimensions)

- *Planning for Access: A Guide for Planning and Modifying Your Home*
- *Programs of EPVA* (a summary of fifteen programs designed to improve the lives of spinal cord injured veterans and people with disabilities)

GENERAL PUBLICATIONS

- *Inside MS*—A quarterly magazine for members of the National Multiple Sclerosis Society (733 Third Avenue, New York, NY 10017; 800-FIGHT-MS.

- *Mainstream*—A monthly magazine available from Exploding Myths, Inc. (2973 Beech Street, San Diego, CA 92101; 619-234-3138)

- *MessageS*—A newsletter sponsored by an unrestricted grant from Berlex Laboratories) available at no cost from Phase Five Communications (114 Fifth Avenue, NY, NY 10011; FAX 212-866-3271)

- *Multiple Sclerosis Quarterly Report*—A quarterly publication with articles on medical management, living with MS, and summaries of research on the cause and treatment of MS, available on a subscription basis from Demos Vermande (386 Park Avenue South, Suite 201, New York, NY 10016; 800-532-8663)

- *A Positive Approach*—A magazine available from A Positive Approach, Inc., a non-profit organization that services individuals with disabilities (P.O. Box 910, Millville, NJ 08322; 609-451-4777)

- *Real Living with MS*—A monthly newsletter available by subscription from the Cobb Group (9420 Bunsen Parkway, Louisville, KY 40220; 800-223-8720)

- *The Very Special Traveler*—A bimonthly newsletter for people with disabilities who travel, published by Beverly Nelson (The Very Special Traveler, P.O. Box 756, New Windsor, MD 21776-9016; 410-635-2881)

- *'We're Accessible': News for Disabled Travelers*—A newsletter from British Columbia for world travelers with disabilities (Lynne Atkinson, 32-1675 Cypress St., Vancouver, B.C. V6J 3L4; 604-731-2197)

Resource Guide*

There is a vast array of resources available to help you in your efforts to meet the challenges of multiple sclerosis. This list is by no means a complete one; it is designed as a starting point in your efforts to identify the resources you need. Each resource that you investigate will lead you to others and they, in turn, will lead you to even more.

INFORMATION SOURCES

CANADIAN REHABILITATION COUNCIL FOR THE DISABLED (CRCD) (45 Sheppard Avenue East, Suite 801, Toronto, Ontario M2N 5W9, Canada; tel: 416-250-7490). The Council is a federation of regional and provincial groups serving individuals with disabilities throughout Canada. It operates an information service and publishes a newsletter and a quarterly journal.

HEALTHTALK INTERACTIVE (800-335-2500). An MS education network is available twenty-four hours a day, providing various kinds of information, including answers to commonly asked questions, a replay of a recent "Living with MS" live broadcast, and presentations on various aspects of symptom management.

---

* This resource list addresses the specific needs of newly diagnosed people with MS. It is a brief version of the comprehensive resource list in *Multiple Sclerosis: The Questions You Have – The Answers You Need;* see " Additional Readings" for details.

INFORMATION CENTER AND LIBRARY, NATIONAL MULTIPLE SCLEROSIS SOCIETY (733 Third Avenue, New York, NY 10017; tel: 800-FIGHT-MS). The Center will answer questions and send you publications of the Society as well as copies of published articles on any topics related to MS.

NATIONAL HEALTH INFORMATION CENTER (P.O. Box 1133, Washington, D.C. 20013; tel: 800-336-4797). The Center maintains a library and a database of health-related organizations. It also provides referrals related to health issues for consumers and professionals.

ELECTRONIC INFORMATION SOURCES

One of the most flexible ways to obtain information on multiple sclerosis is by using a computer and a modem. It is possible to dial a number of services that provide access to information about MS. These include the "big three" online services - America OnLine, CompuServe, and Prodigy (see below for customer service numbers). If you are not currently a subscriber and would like information on how to join, call one or more of these numbers. If you are a subscriber, you can access information about MS by entering one of the commands listed below.

Some of these sources of information are available only if you are a subscriber to the service. However, there are also many sources of information available free through the Internet on the World Wide Web. For example, the National Multiple Sclerosis Society has a home page on the World Wide Web at: http://www.nmss.org/. The other sources of MS information on the World Wide Web are too numerous to list. If you are an experienced "net surfer," switch to your favorite search facility and enter the keywords "MS" or "multiple sclerosis." This will generally give you a listing of dozens of web sites that pertain to MS. Keep in mind, however, that the World Wide Web is a free and open medium; while many of the web sites have excellent and useful information, others may contain highly unusual and inaccurate information.

- *America OnLine:* 800-827-6364 (GO TO NMSS).
- *CompuServe:* 800-487-6227 (GO MULTSCLER).
- *Prodigy:* 800-776-3449 (JUMP MS FORUM).

On the Internet: Access USENET NEWSGROUP-ALT.SUPPORT.MULT-SCLEROSIS.

RESOURCE MATERIALS

COMPLETE DRUG REFERENCE. (Compiled by United States Pharmacopoeia, published by Consumer Report Books, A division of Consumers Union, Yonkers, NY.). This comprehensive, readable, and easy-to-use drug reference includes almost every prescription and non-prescription medication available in the United States and Canada. A new edition is published yearly.

AGENCIES AND ORGANIZATIONS

CONSORTIUM OF MULTIPLE SCLEROSIS CENTERS (CMSC) (c/o Gimbel MS Center at Holy Name Hospital, 718 Teaneck Road, Teaneck, NJ 07666; tel: 201-837-0727). The CMSC is made up of numerous MS centers throughout the United States and Canada. The Consortium's mission is to disseminate information to clinicians, increase resources and opportunities for research, and advance the standard of care for multiple sclerosis. The CMSC is a multidisciplinary organization, bringing together health care professionals from many fields involved in MS patient care. Department of Veterans Affairs (VA) (810 Vermont Avenue, N.W., Washington, D.C. 20420; tel: 202-328-5198). The VA provides a wide range of benefits and services to those who have served in the armed forces, their dependents, beneficiaries of deceased veterans, and dependent children of veterans with severe disabilities.

EASTERN PARALYZED VETERANS ASSOCIATION (EPVA) (75-20 Astoria Boulevard, Jackson Heights, NY 11370; tel: 718-803-EPVA). EPVA is a private, non-profit organization dedicated to serving the needs of its members as well as other people with disabilities. While offering a wide range of benefits to member veterans with spinal cord dysfunction (including hospital liaison, sports and recreation, wheelchair repair, adaptive architectural consultations, research and educational services, communications, and library and information services, they will also provide brochures and information on a variety of subjects, free of charge to the general public (see "Additional Readings").

NATIONAL MULTIPLE SCLEROSIS SOCIETY (NMSS) (733 Third Avenue, New York, NY 10017; tel: 800-FIGHT-MS). The NMSS funds both basic and health services research. An office of professional education programs maintains a speakers' bureau and supports professional education programs both nationally and in the individual chapters. Over 140 chapters and branches of the Society provide direct services to people with MS and their families to meet their MS-related needs and improve quality of life. Services include information and referral, counseling, equipment loan, and social and recreational support programs. The National Office will put you in touch with your closest chapter. The Information Resource Center and Library is available to answer questions and provide a wide range of educational materials, as well as reprints of articles written about MS.

PARALYZED VETERANS OF AMERICA (PVA) (801 Eighteenth Street, N.W., Washington, D.C., 20006; tel: 202-USA-1300). PVA provides extensive services to veterans; members increasingly include those diagnosed with multiple sclerosis.

ASSISTIVE TECHNOLOGY

NATIONAL REHABILITATION INFORMATION CENTER (NARIC) (8455 Colesville Road, Silver Spring, MD 20910; tel: 800-346-2742; 301-588-9284; fax: 301-587-1967). NARIC is a library and information center on disability and rehabilitation, funded by the National Institute on Disability and Rehabilitation Research (NIDRR). NARIC operates two databases—ABLEDATA and REHABDATA. NARIC collects and disseminates the results of federally funded research projects and has a collection that includes commercially published books, journal articles, and audiovisual materials. NARIC is committed to serving both professionals and consumers who are interested in disability and rehabilitation. Information specialists can answer simple information requests and provide referrals immediately and at no cost. More complex database searches are available at nominal cost.

ABLEDATA (8455 Colesville Road Suite 935, Silver Spring, MD 20910; tel: 301-588-9284; 800-227-0216; fax: 301-589-3563. ABLEDATA is a national database of information on assistive technology designed to enable persons with disabilities to identify and locate the devices that will assist them in their home, work, and leisure activities. Information specialists are available to answer questions during regular business hours. ABLE INFORM BBS is available twenty-four hours a day to customers with a computer, modem, and telecommunications software.

REHABDATA (8455 Colesville Road, Suite 935, Silver Spring, MD 20910; tel: 301-588-9284; 800-346-2742) REHABDATA is a database containing bibliographic records with abstracts and summaries of the materials contained in the NARIC (National Rehabilitation Information Information Center) library of disability rehabilitation materials. Information specialists are available to conduct a database search on any rehabilitation related topic.

TRAVEL

DIRECTORY OF TRAVEL AGENCIES FOR THE DISABLED. (Written by Helen Hecker, published by Twin Peaks Press, P.O. Box 129, Vancouver, WA 98666-0129). This directory lists travel agents who specialize in arranging travel plans for people with disabilities.

INFORMATION FOR HANDICAPPED TRAVELERS (available free of charge from the National Library Service for the Blind and Physically Handicapped, 1291 Taylor Street, N.W., Washington, D.C. 20542; tel: 800-424-8567; 202-707-5100). A booklet providing information about travel agents, transportation, and information centers for individuals with disabilities.

WILDERNESS INQUIRY (1313 5th Street, S.E., Box 84, Minneapolis, MN 55414; tel: 800-728-0719; 612-379-3858). Wilderness Inquiry sponsors trips into the wilderness for people with disabilities or chronic conditions.

PUBLISHING COMPANIES SPECIALIZING IN HEALTH AND DISABILITY ISSUES

DEMOS VERMANDE (386 Park Avenue South, Suite 201, New York, NY 10016; tel: 800-532-8663).

RESOURCES FOR REHABILITATION (33 Bedford Street, Suite 19A, Lexington, MA 02173; tel: 617-862-6455).

TWIN PEAKS PRESS (P.O. Box 129, Vancouver, WA 98666; tel: 800-637-2256).

WOODBINE HOUSE (Publishers of the Special-Needs Collection) (6510 Bells Mill Road, Bethesda, MD 20817; tel: 301-897-3570; 800-843-7323).

Index